Laughter is the Best Medicine: Book of Medical Cartoons

Featuring Cartoons From
Barron's
The New Yorker
The Wall Street Journal
and more!

Front Cover illustration: Charlie Hankin
Back Cover illustration: Charles Barsotti
Introduction: Bob Mankoff
Edited By: Darren Kornblut

Dedicated to Jennifer & Bea

Cartoon Collections, LLC
10 Grand Central, 29th Floor
New York, NY 10017

For cartoon licensing information visit www.cartoonstock.com
Create a personalized version of tis book at www.cartoonstockgifts.com

First edition published 2024

Item # 49237
UPC: 978-1-963079-10-4

Introduction

Welcome to a world where wit and wisdom merge, where laughter intertwines with the complexities of the human body, and where doctors and patients find solace in shared hilarity. Within the pages of this extraordinary collection, we explore the realm of medicine through the eyes of the world's best cartoonists. From the waiting room to the operating theater, from a yearly physical exam to the lab, their pens have transformed the daily dramas of doctors and their patients into moments of levity and insight.

As the former Cartoon Editor of *The New Yorker*, I have long recognized the power of a well-crafted cartoon to capture the essence of our lives. Medicine, with its blend of science, empathy, and even a touch of absurdity, provides a rich tapestry of material for our cartoonists to mine. Within these pages, you will discover an array of brilliant artists who have deftly translated the inherent comedy and pathos of the medical world into moments of visual brilliance.

So, prepare yourself for a journey into the whimsical world of medical cartoons. Let these delightful illustrations and captions guide you through the corridors of hospitals, the pangs of diagnosis, and the triumphs of healing. May these pages bring a smile to your face, lighten your burdens, and remind you that laughter truly is the best medicine.

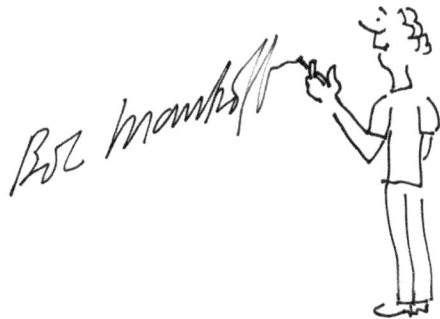

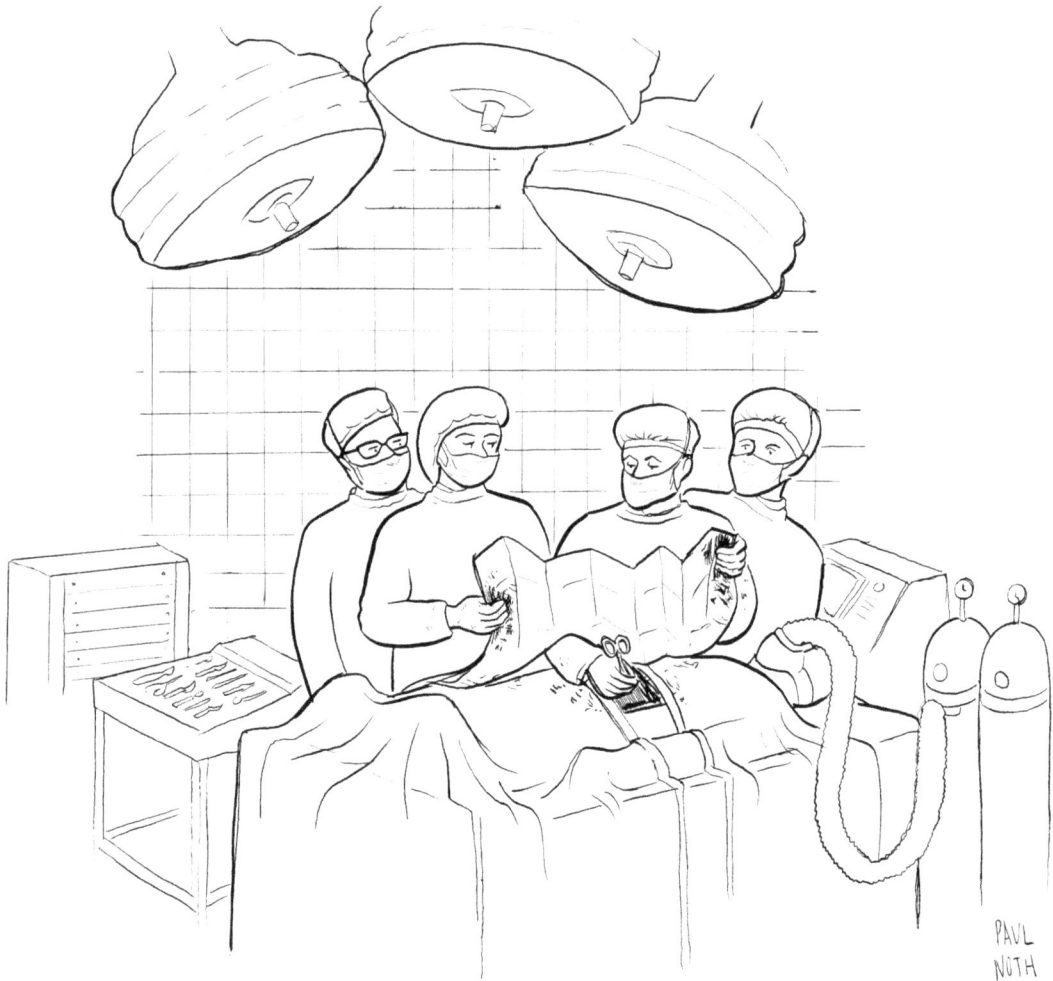

"According to this, we're not even in Mrs. Feldman anymore."

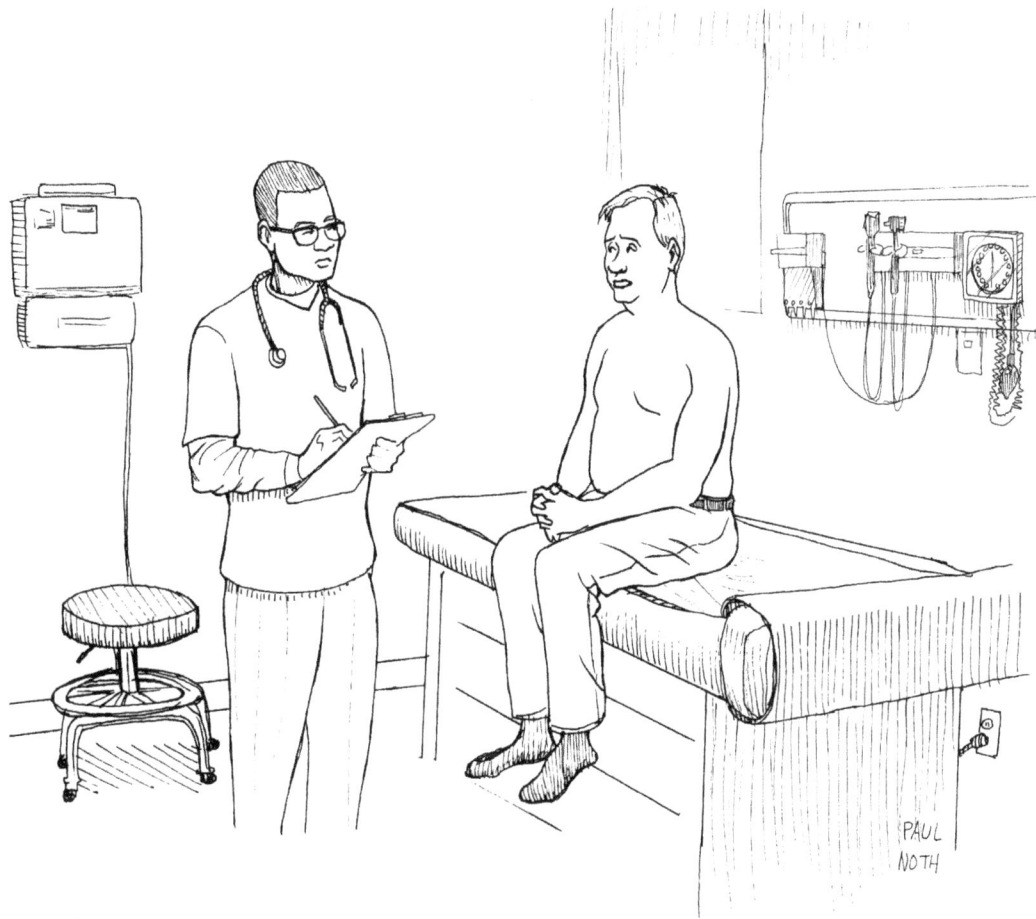

"Will I still be able to not exercise?"

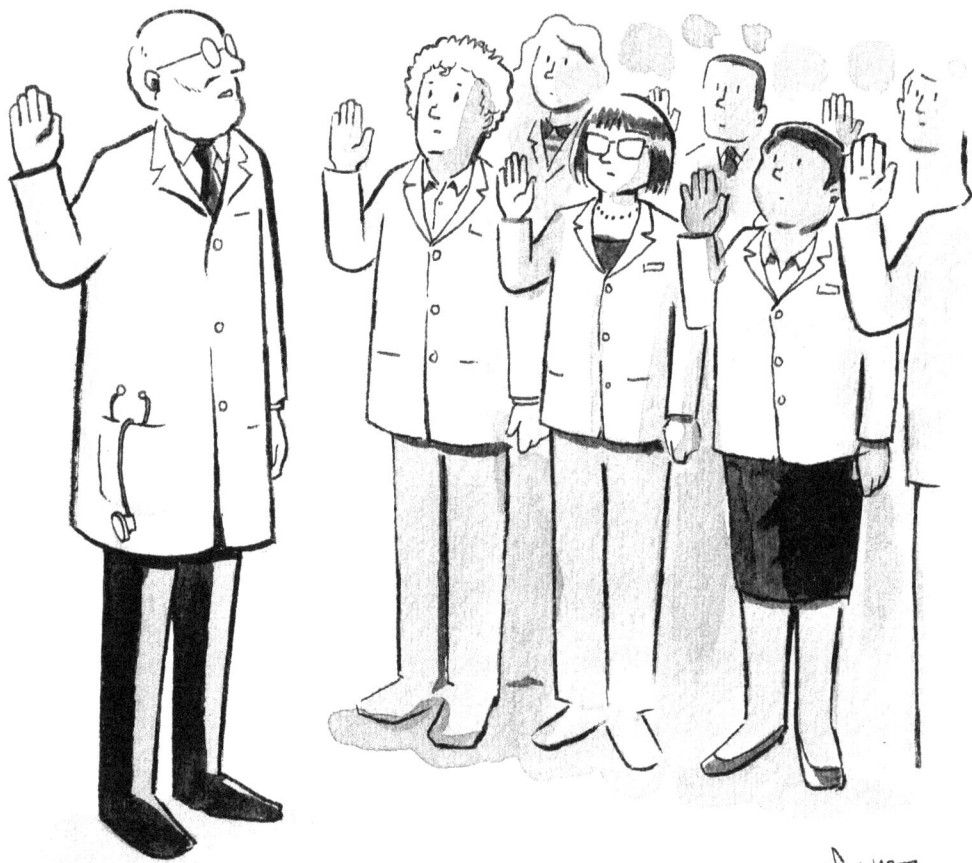

"First, do no harm. After that, go nuts."

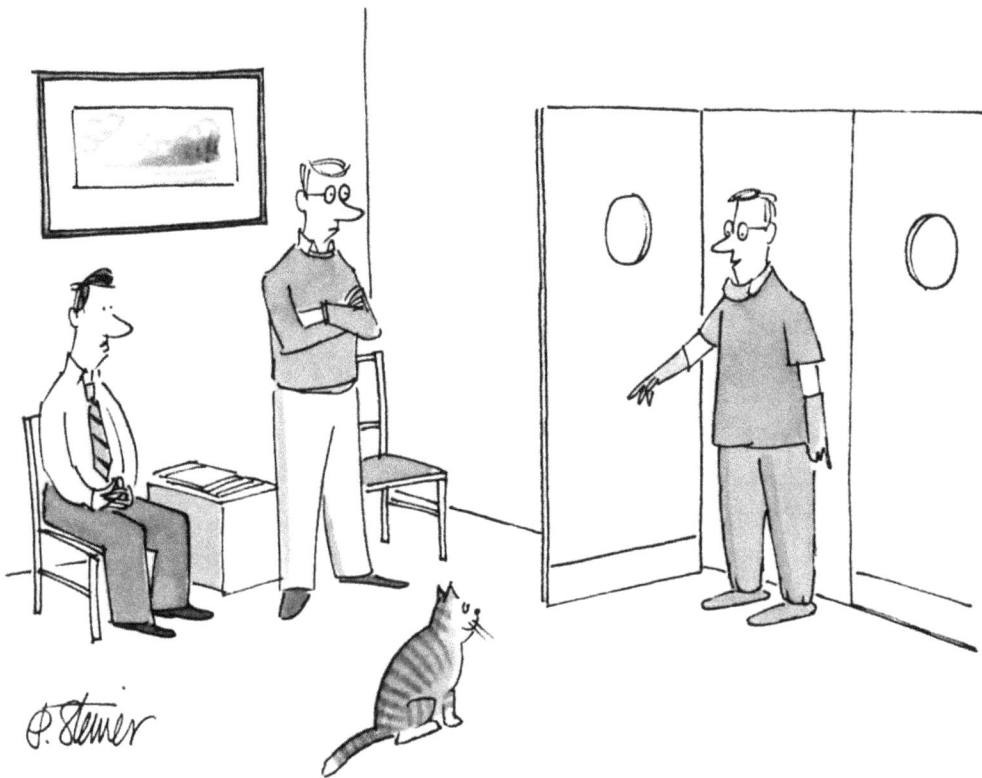

"It's kittens."

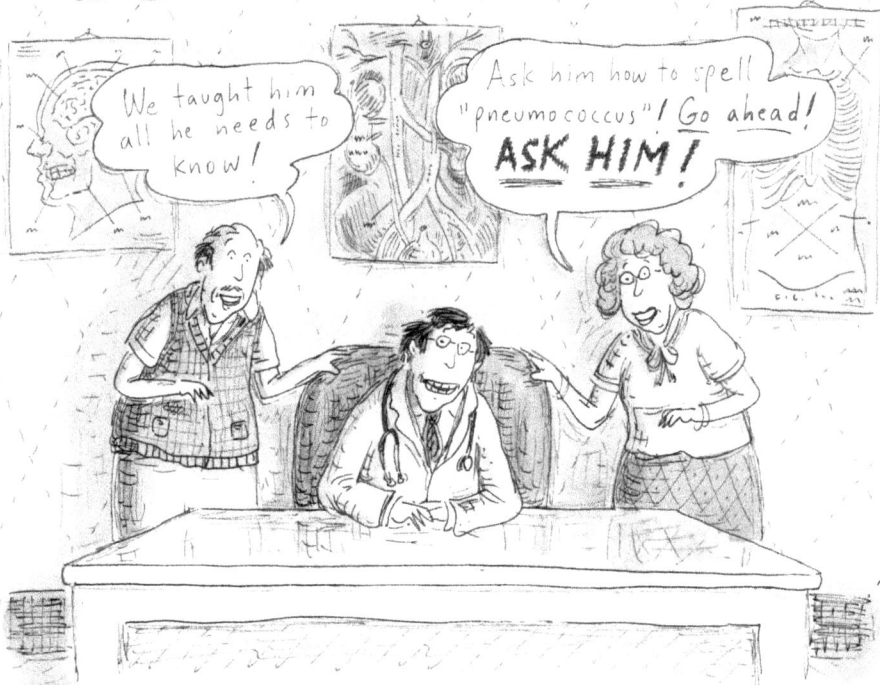

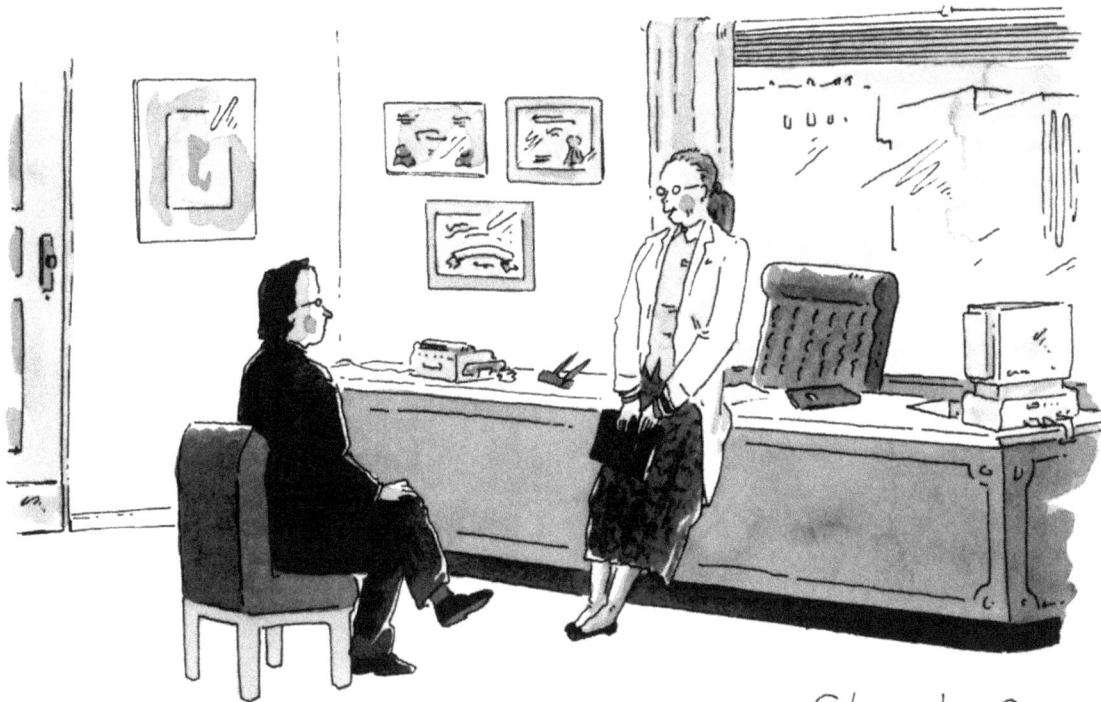

"*Our integrated approach to medicine skillfully combines an array of holistic alternative treatments with a sophisticated computerized billing service.*"

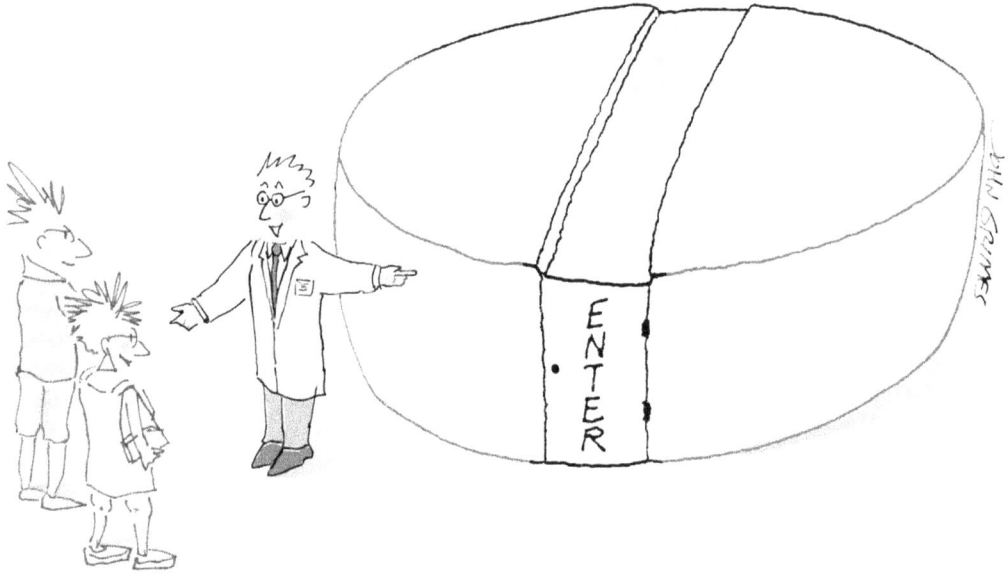

"It's a new kind of pill: It takes <u>you!</u>"

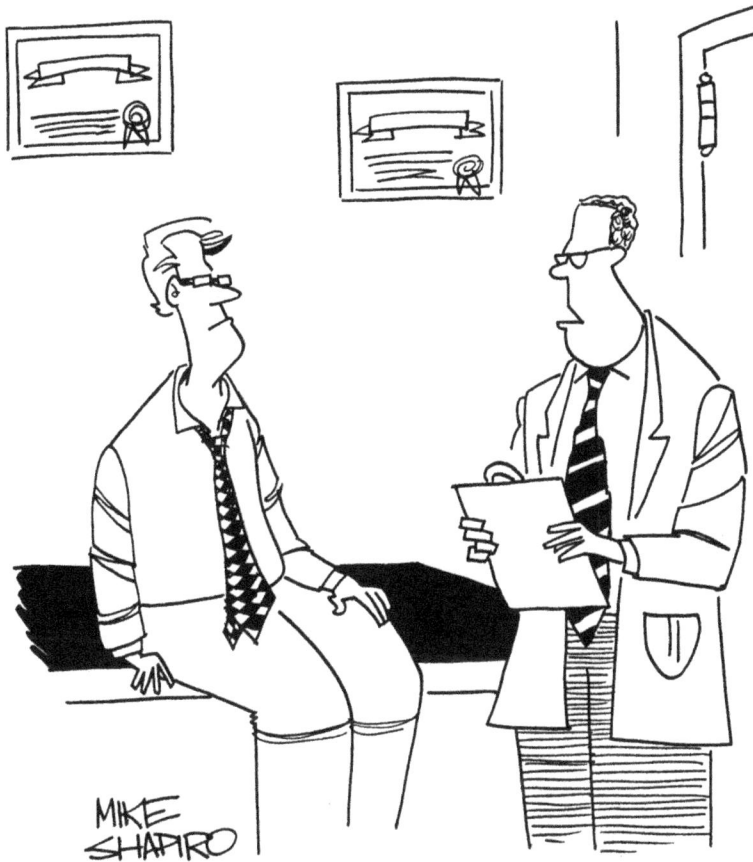

"I find a good way to avoid stress is to close the curtains, climb into bed, and pull the covers over my head."

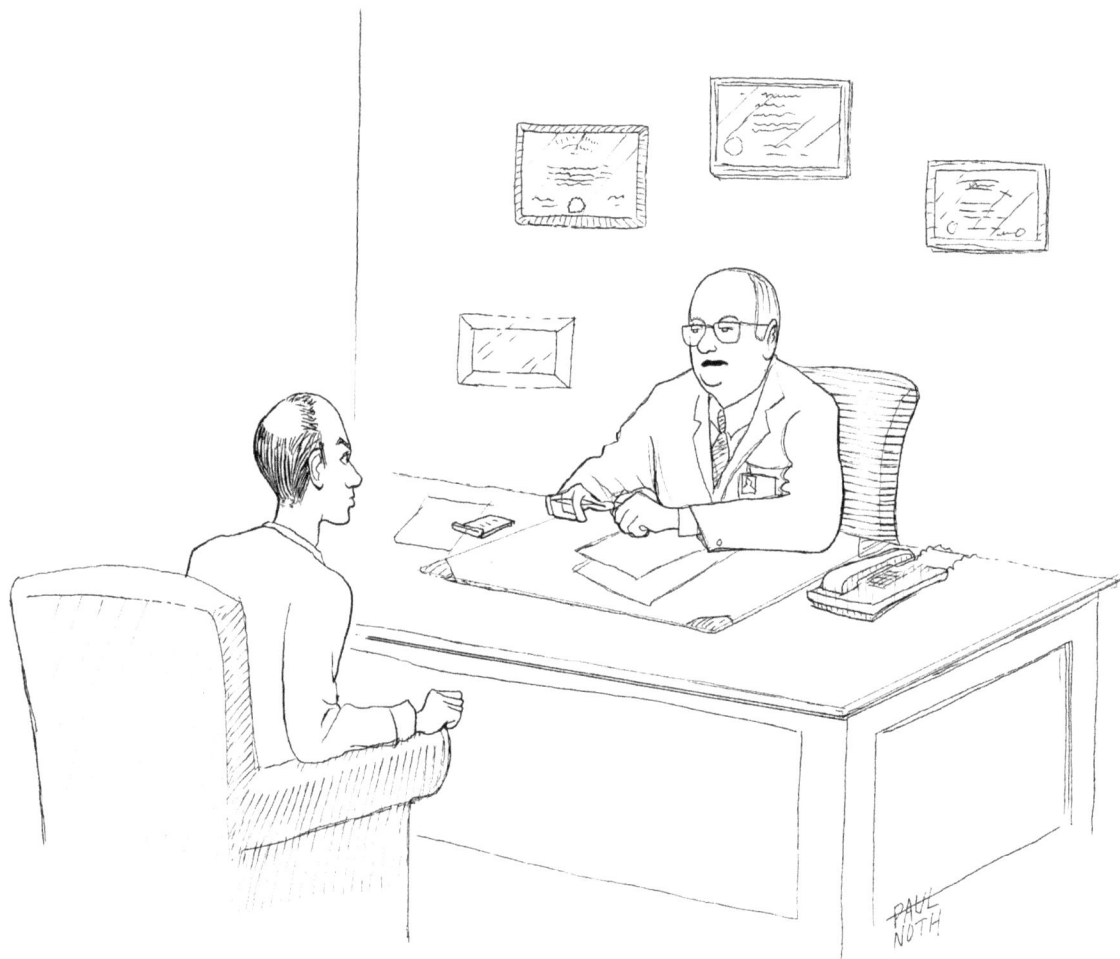

"I'm a doctor—I can add 'ectomy' to any word I choose."

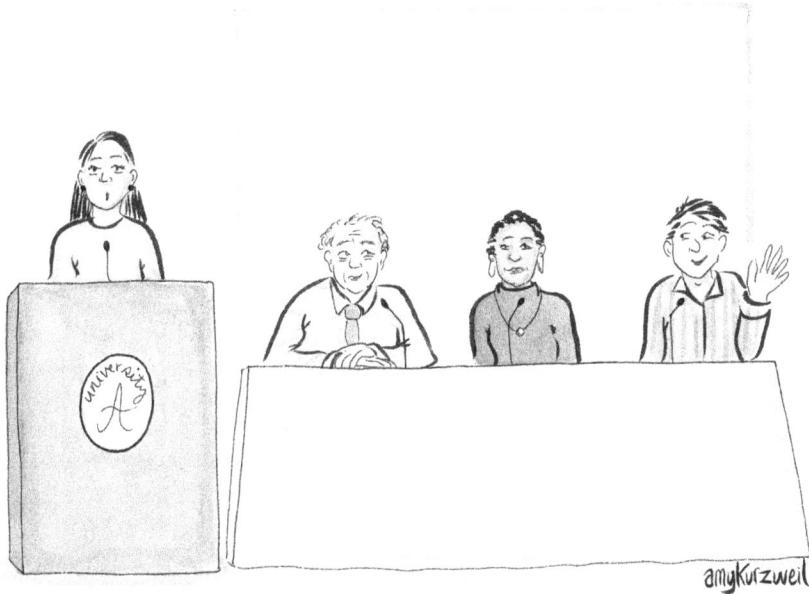

"Our panel of experts includes: Dr. Fiorini, practicing neuroscientist and professor emeritus at Oxford, Dr. Nouveau, professor of psychology at Harvard and author of five critically acclaimed books in her field, and Dan, who has listened to two different podcasts on this topic."

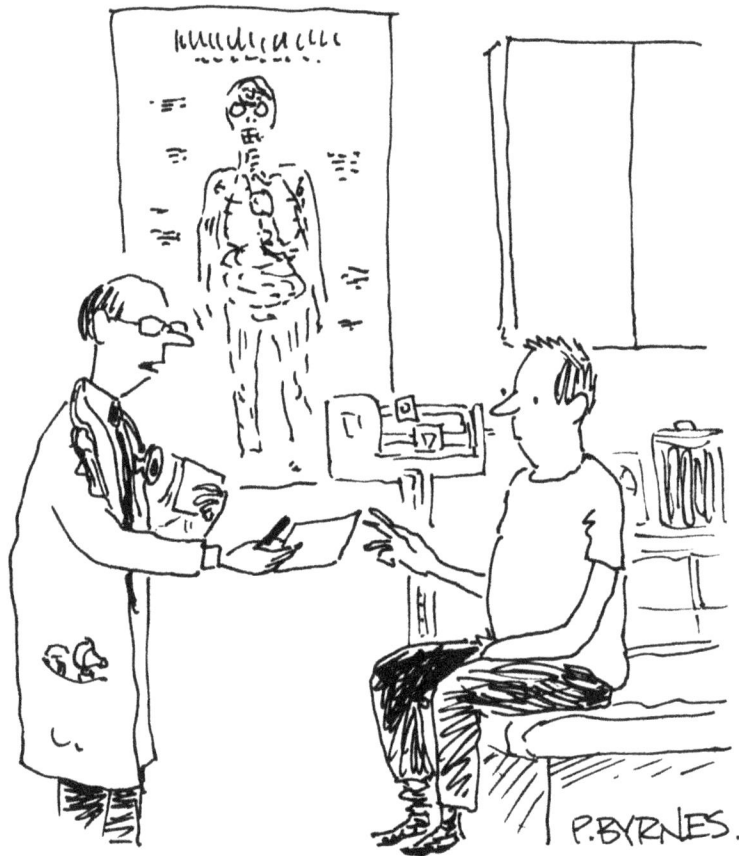

"*For the pain, these have proven to be the most effective swear words.*"

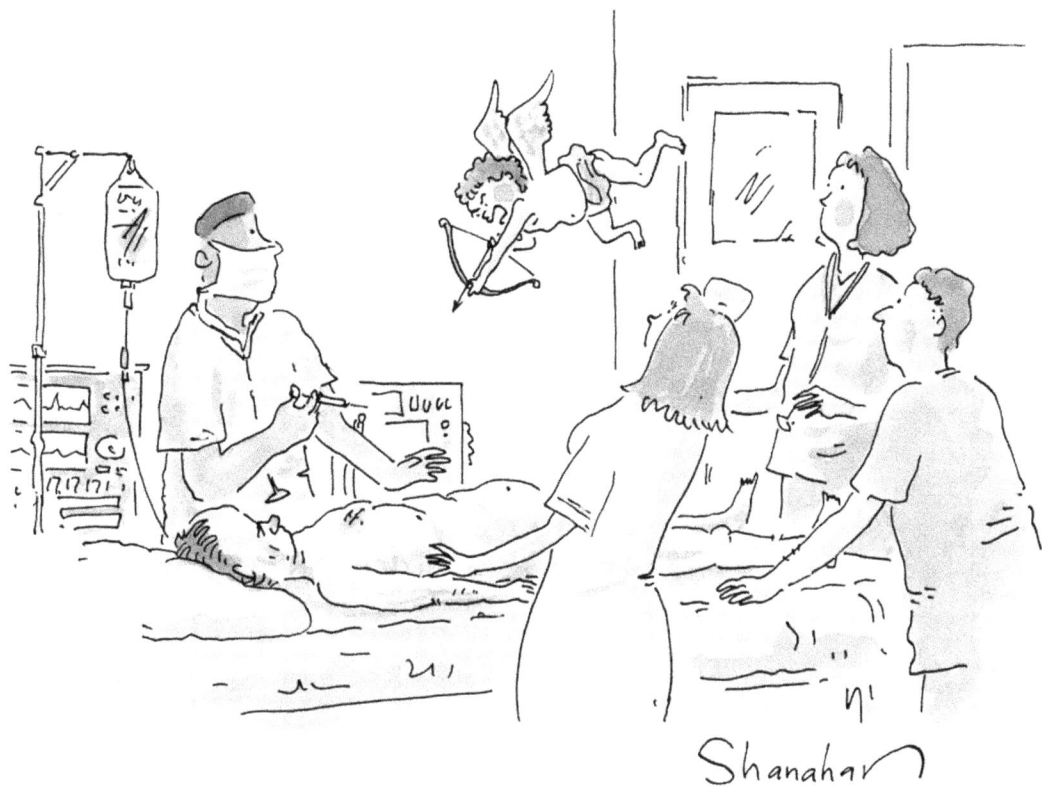

"*Clear!*"

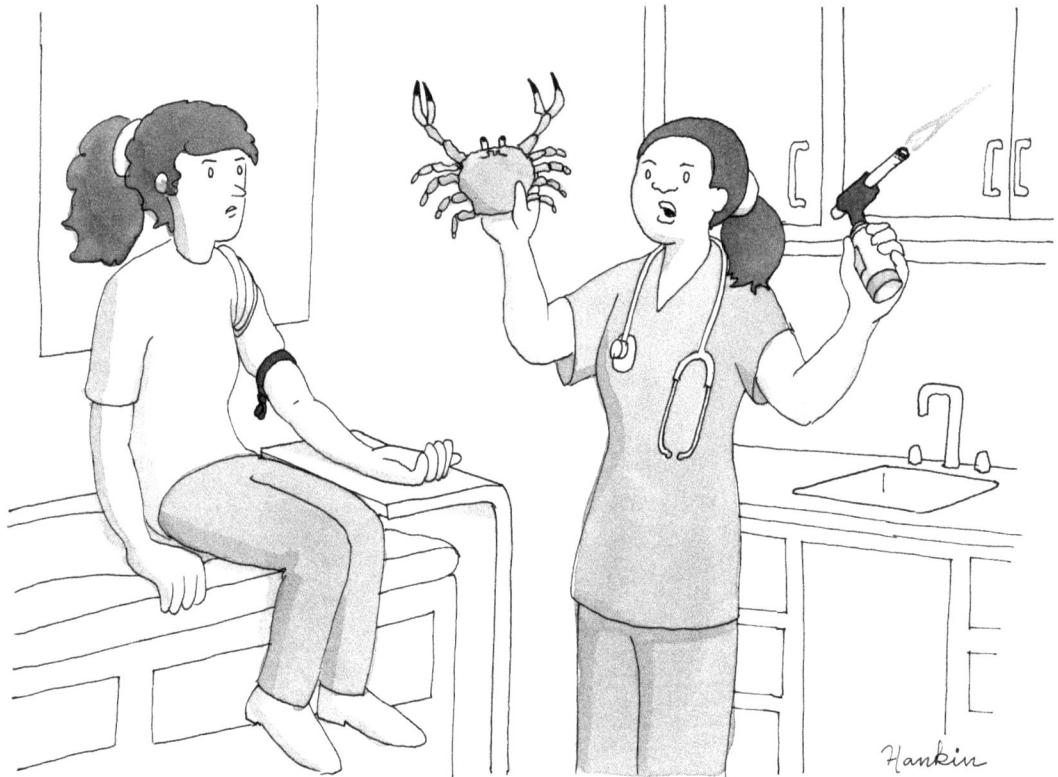

"You'll feel a pinch and then a burn."

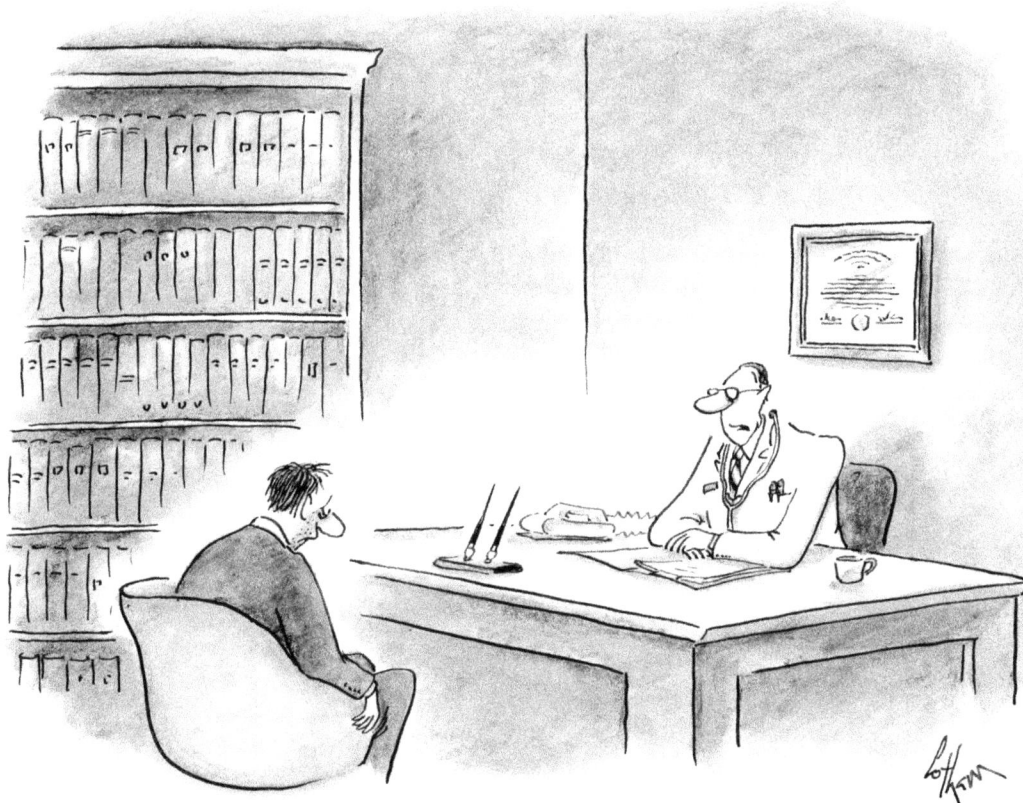

"Unfortunately, there's no cure—not even a race for a cure."

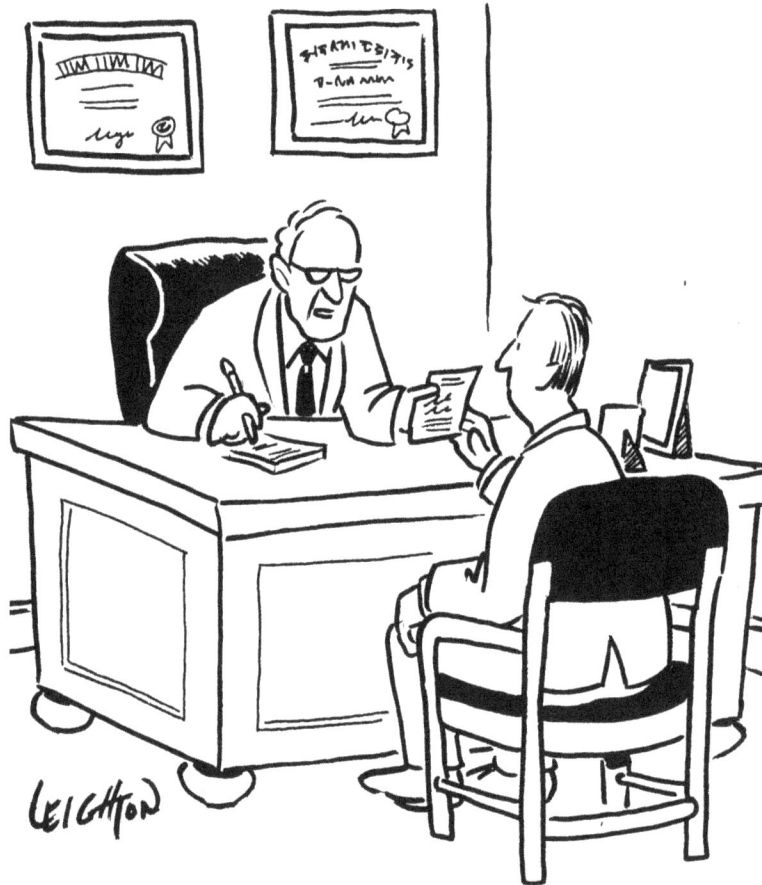

"Now remember, this is an experimental treatment, so have some fun with it."

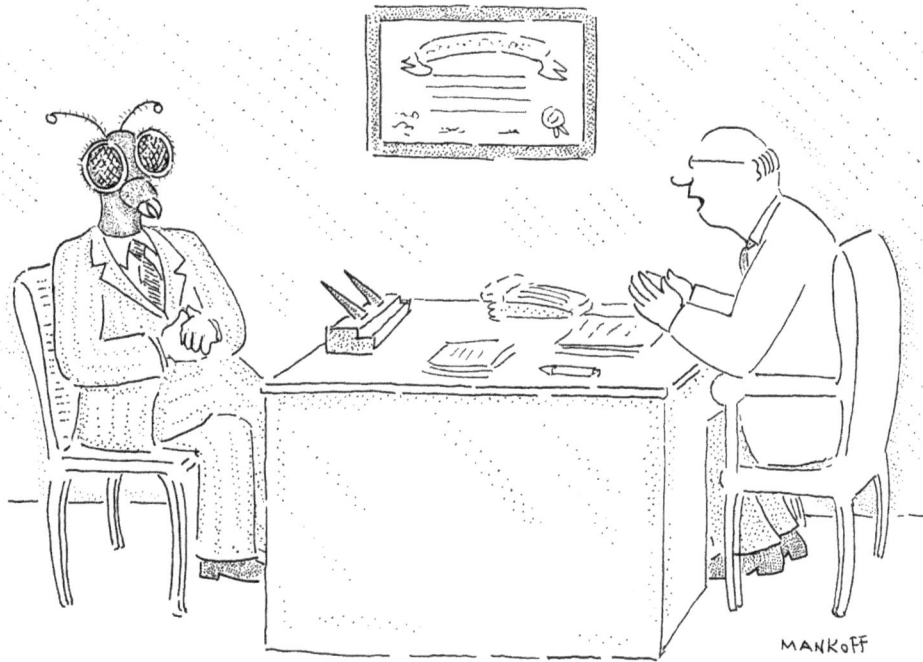

"We think it has something to do with your genome."

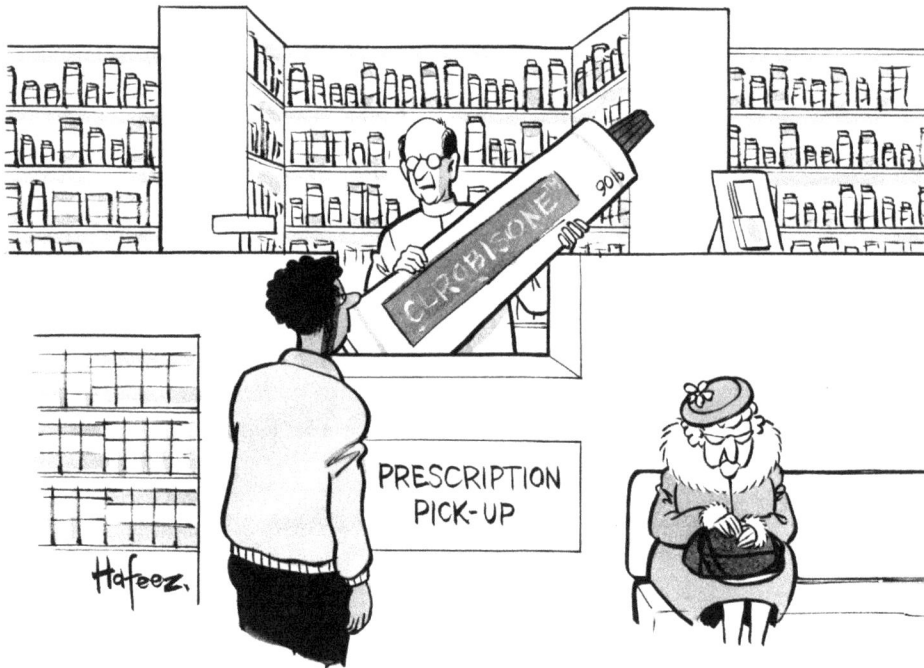

"*Rub this on everything.*"

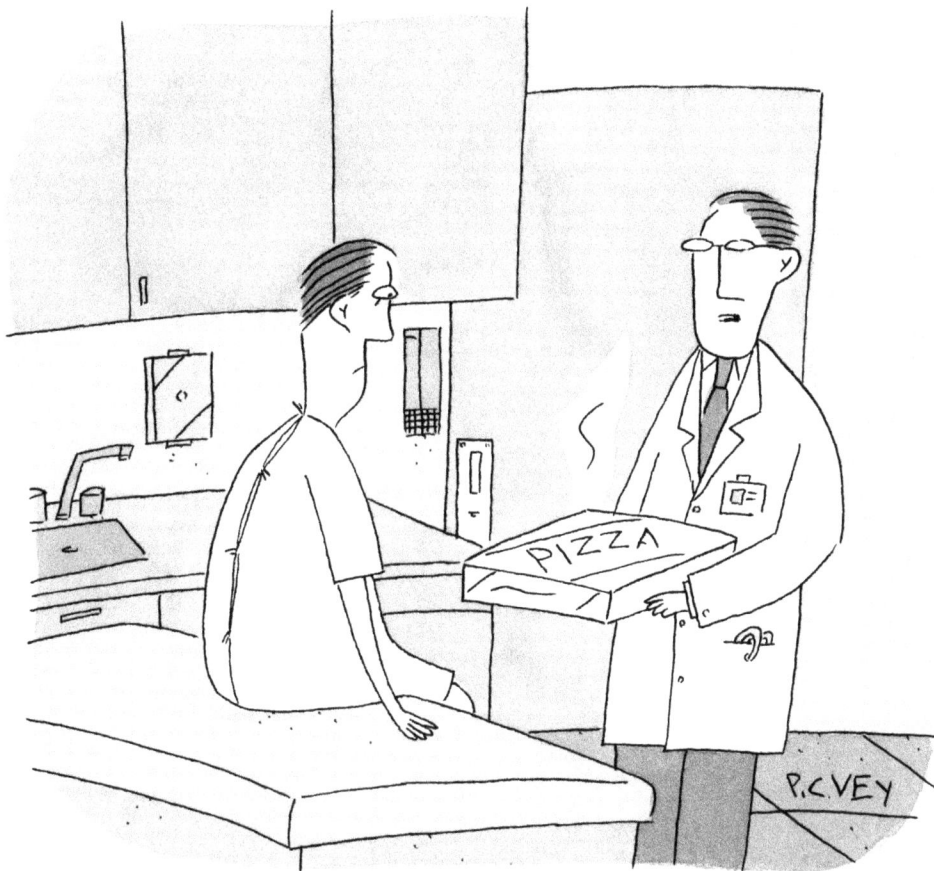

"We find pizza softens the blow of bad news."

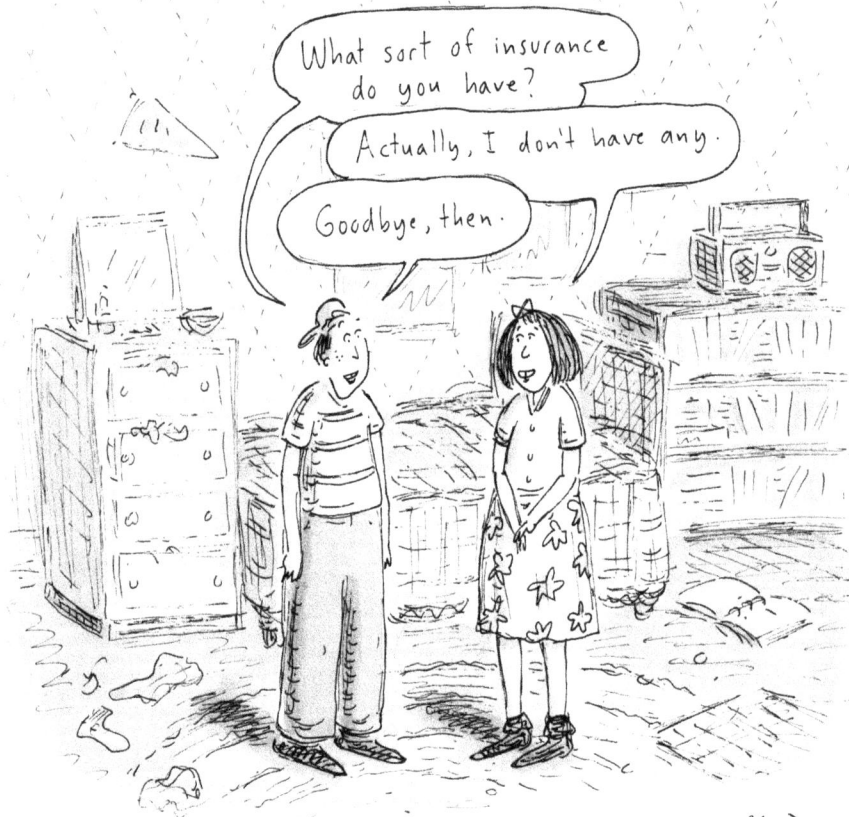

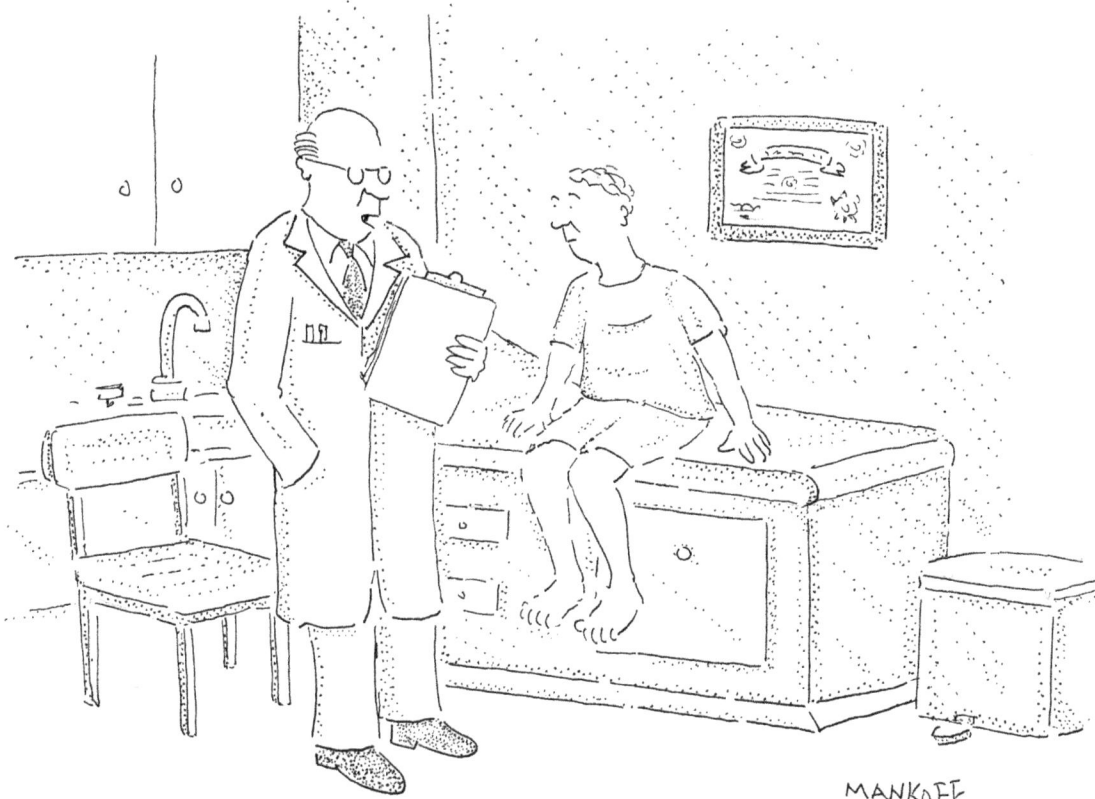

"Uh-oh, your coverage doesn't seem to include illness."

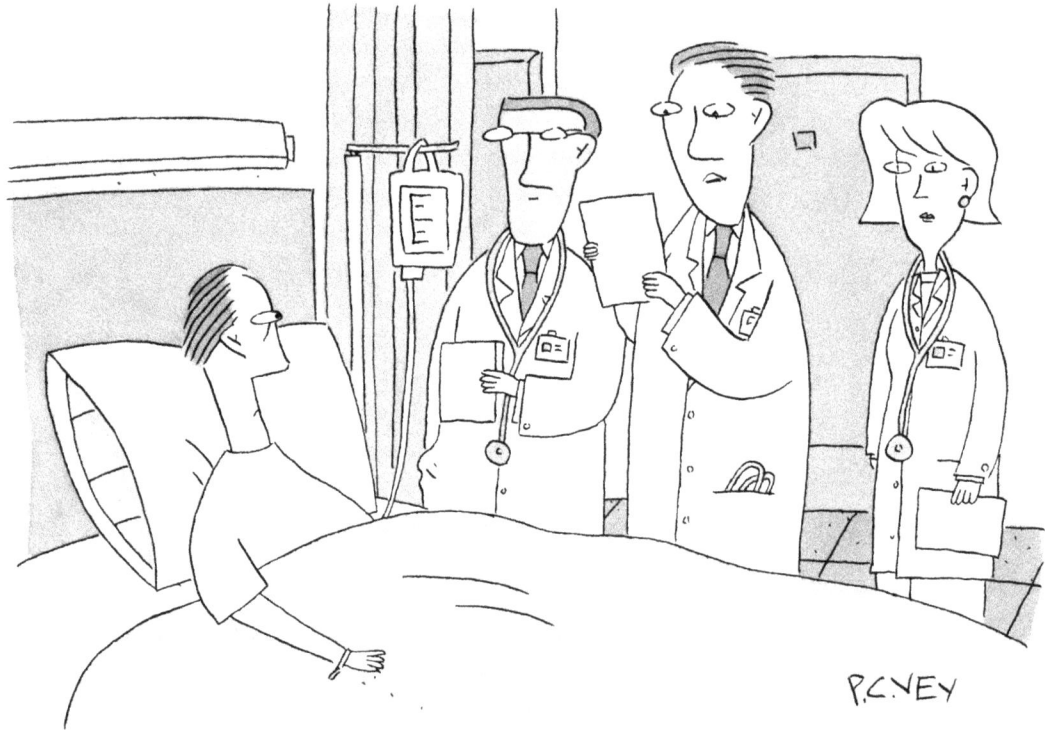

"We'd like to start out being very involved with you but eventually be drawn away to much more interesting cases down the hall."

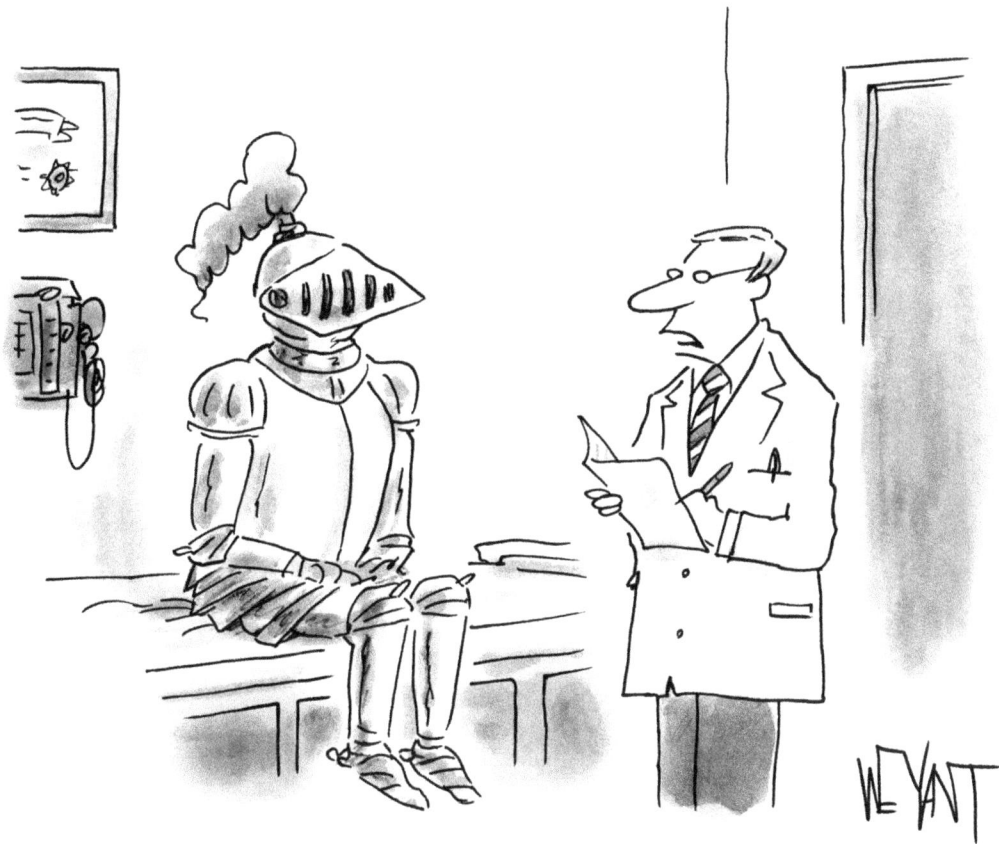

"Are you sure you wouldn't rather just get the vaccine?"

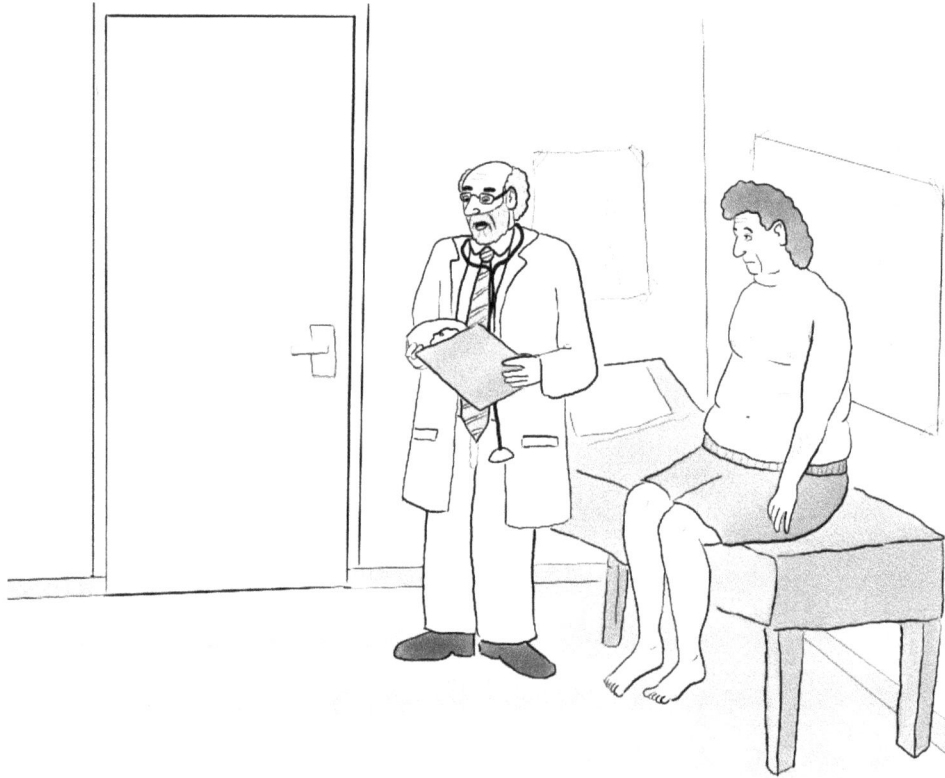

"The good news is you'll have a condition named after you."

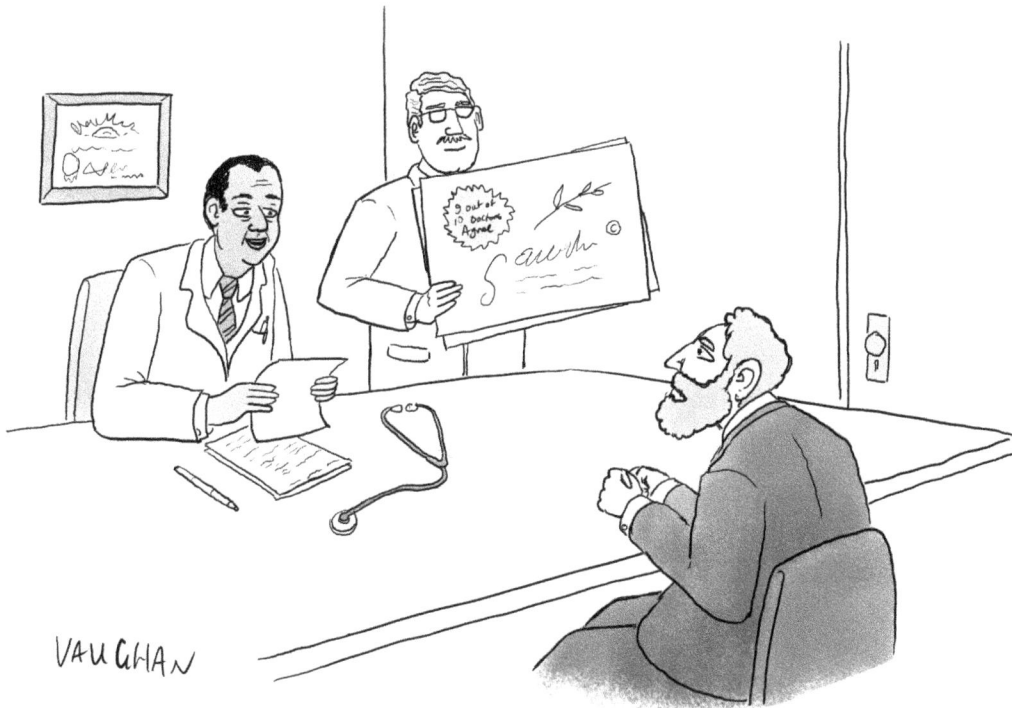

"And we'll find out your test results
right after a word from our sponsors"

1989

2019

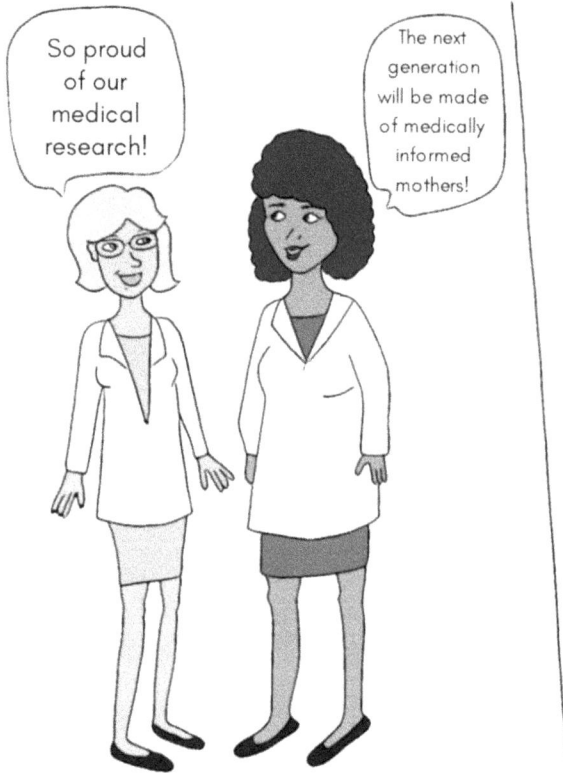

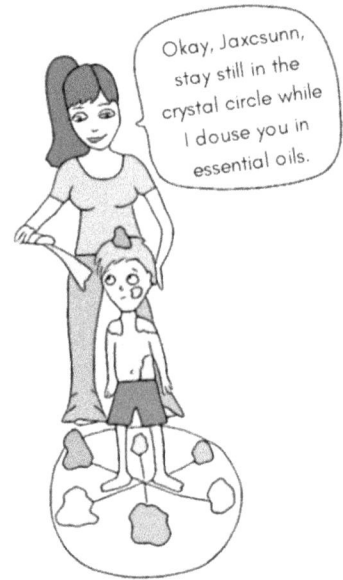

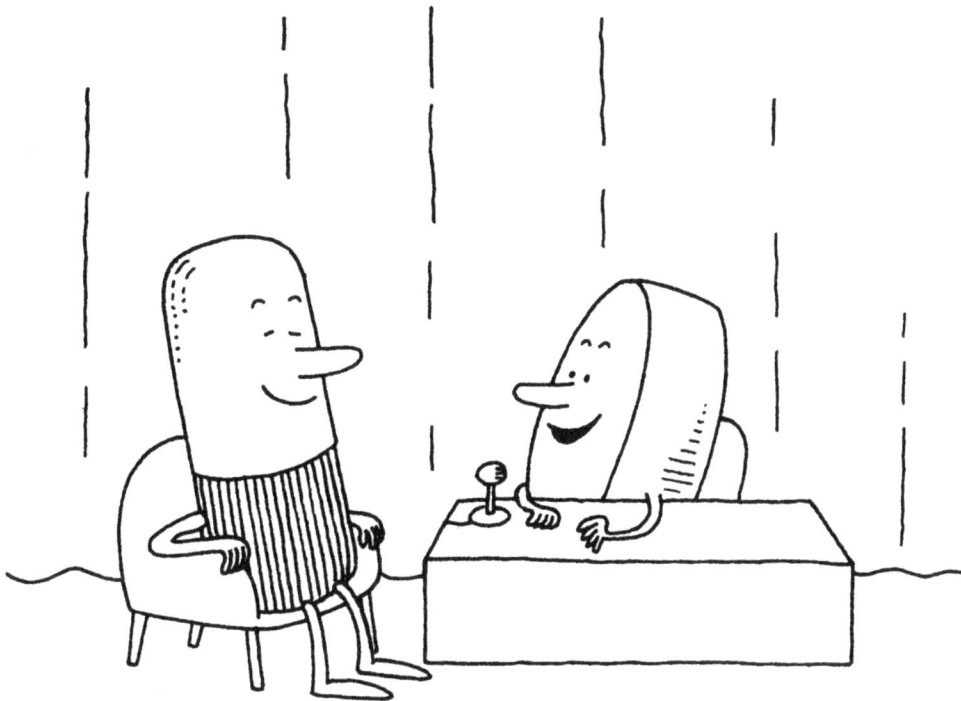

"I understand they've uncovered some weird new side effects since you were here last."

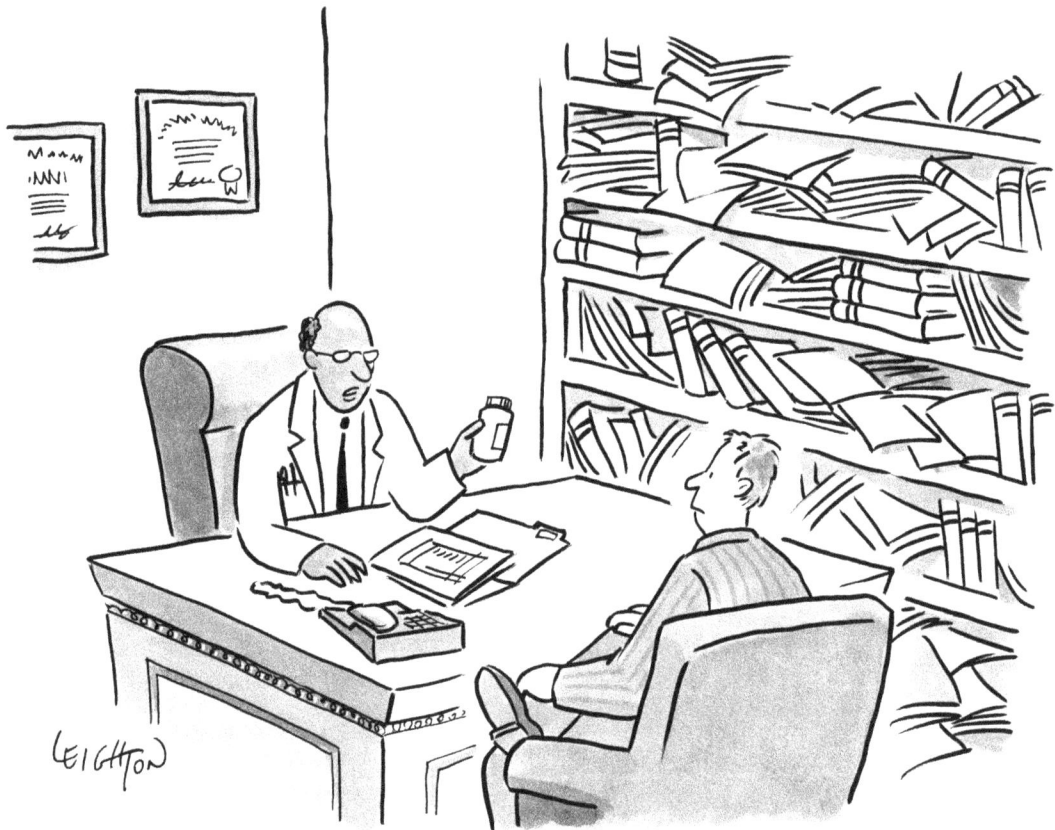

"These pills will cure your O.C.D., but first
I wonder if you could organize my shelves."

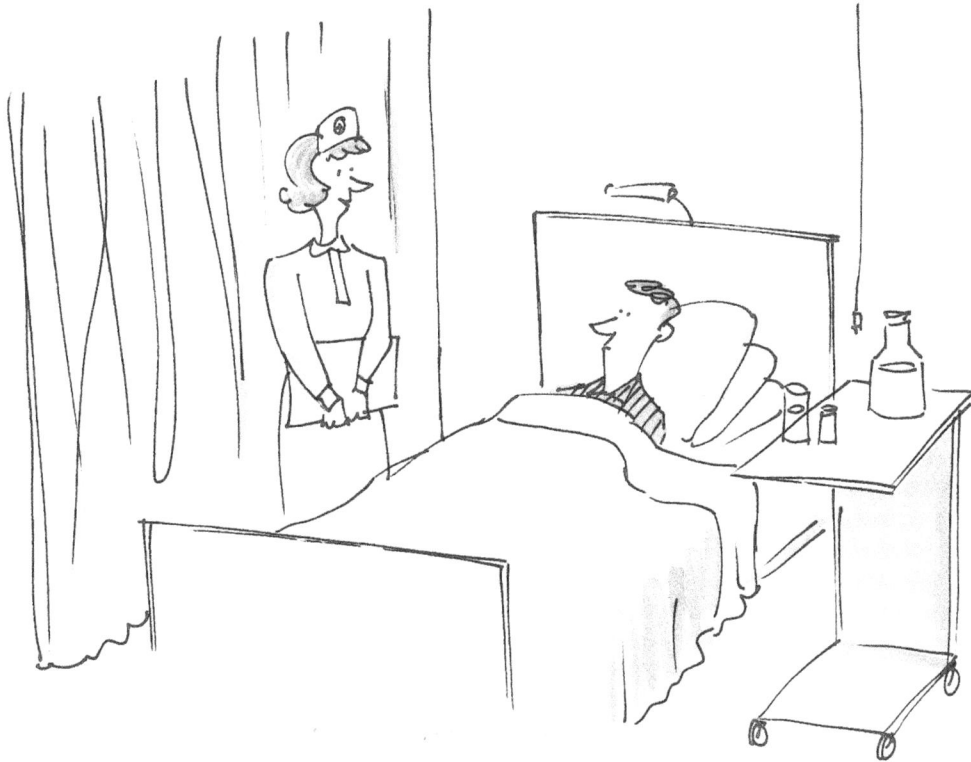

"We're going to run some tests: bloodwork, a cat-scan, and the S.A.T.'s."

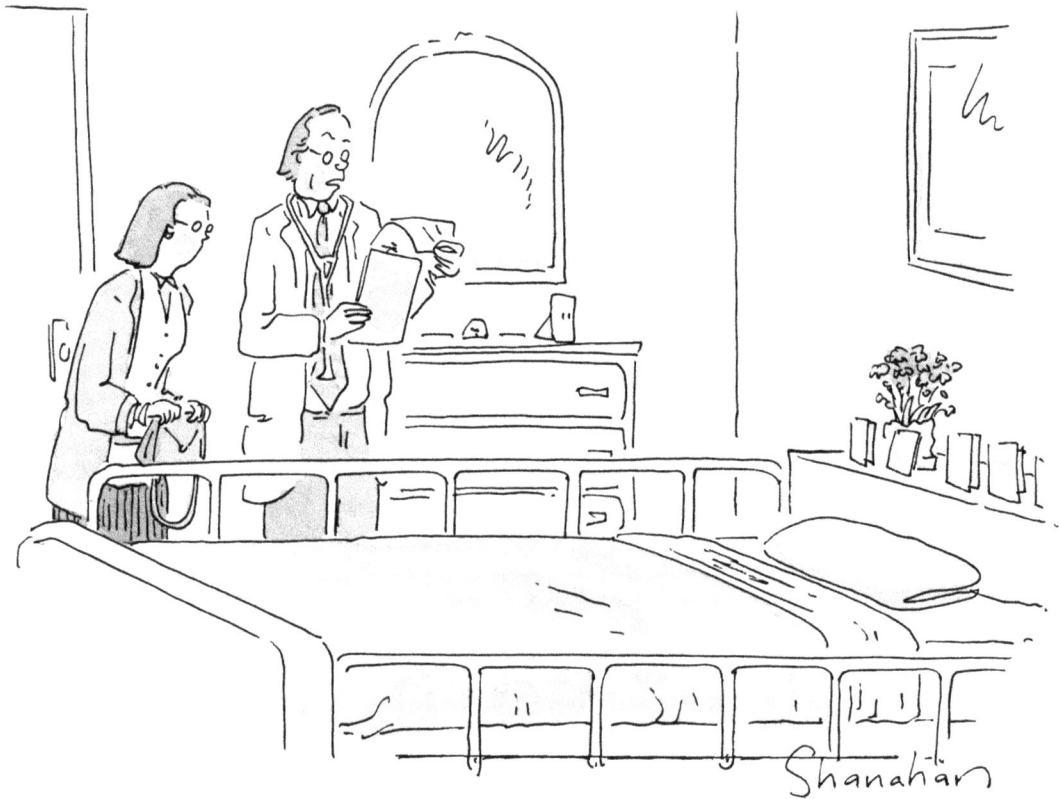

"Good news, Mrs. Bryant – I think we got it all."

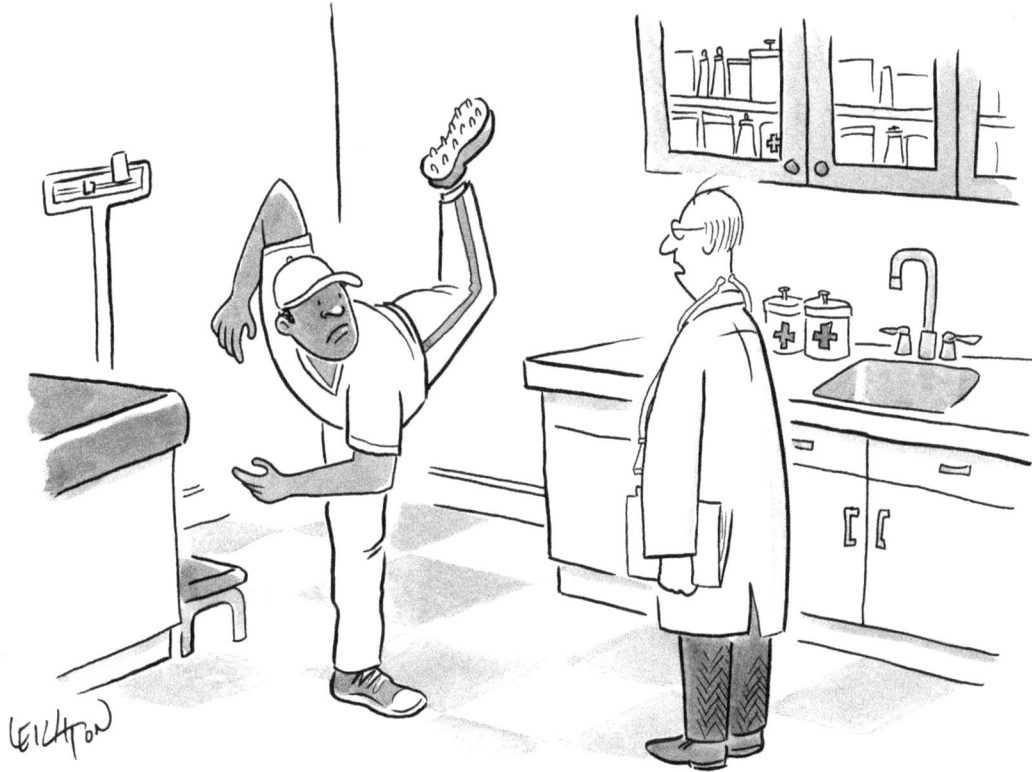

"Then don't do that."

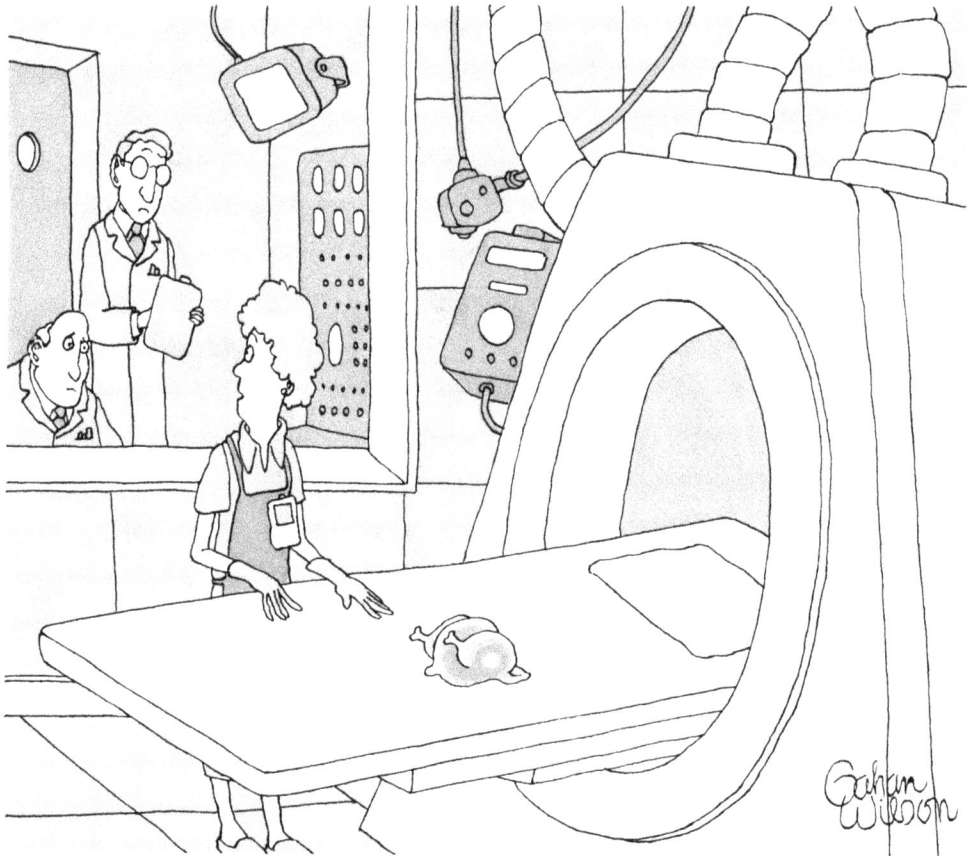

"The machine's done something really weird to Mr. Hendrickson."

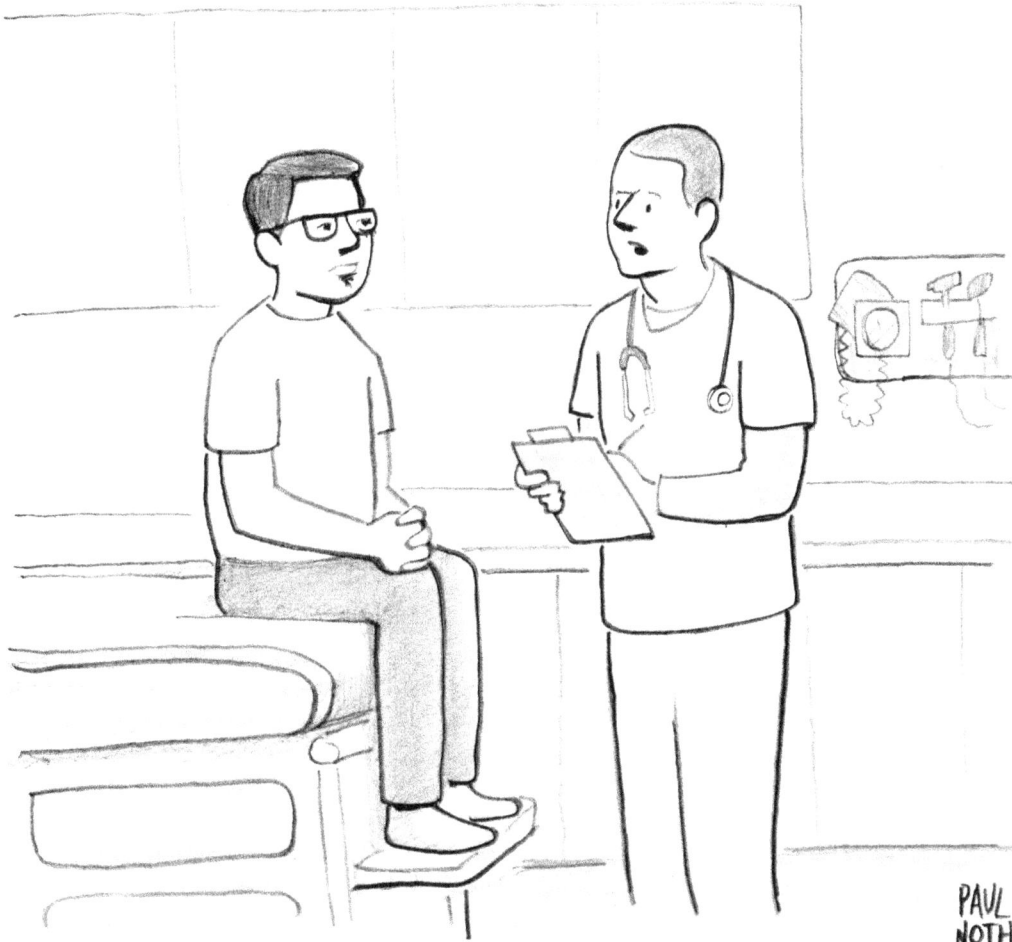

"It's a soul patch, but luckily we've caught it early."

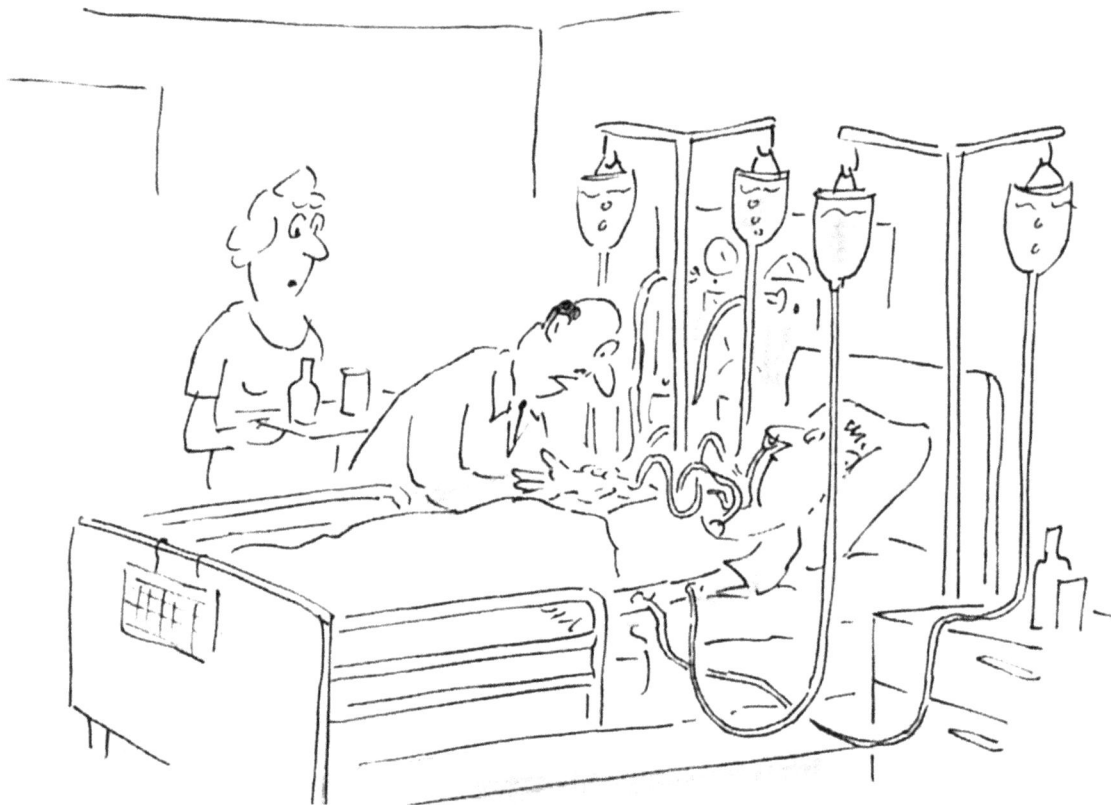

"Good heavens! Who hooked you up? This one is cable TV!"

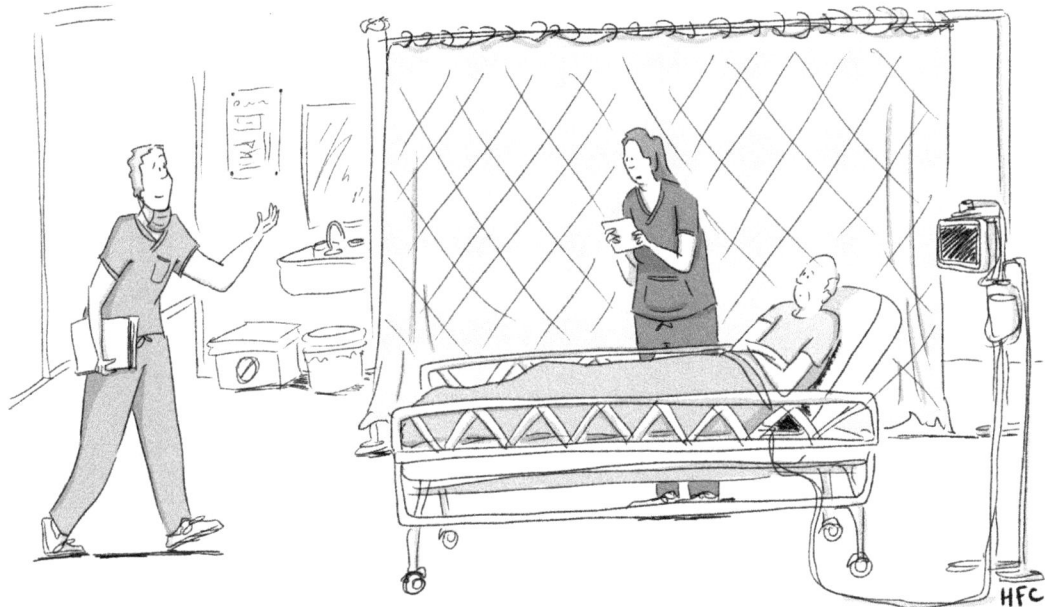

"You may know him from his short time in the waiting room, or his recent works 'Prior Authorization' and 'Prescription Refills'. He was named 'A recent missed call' in your phone just last week. Here he is, your doctor!"

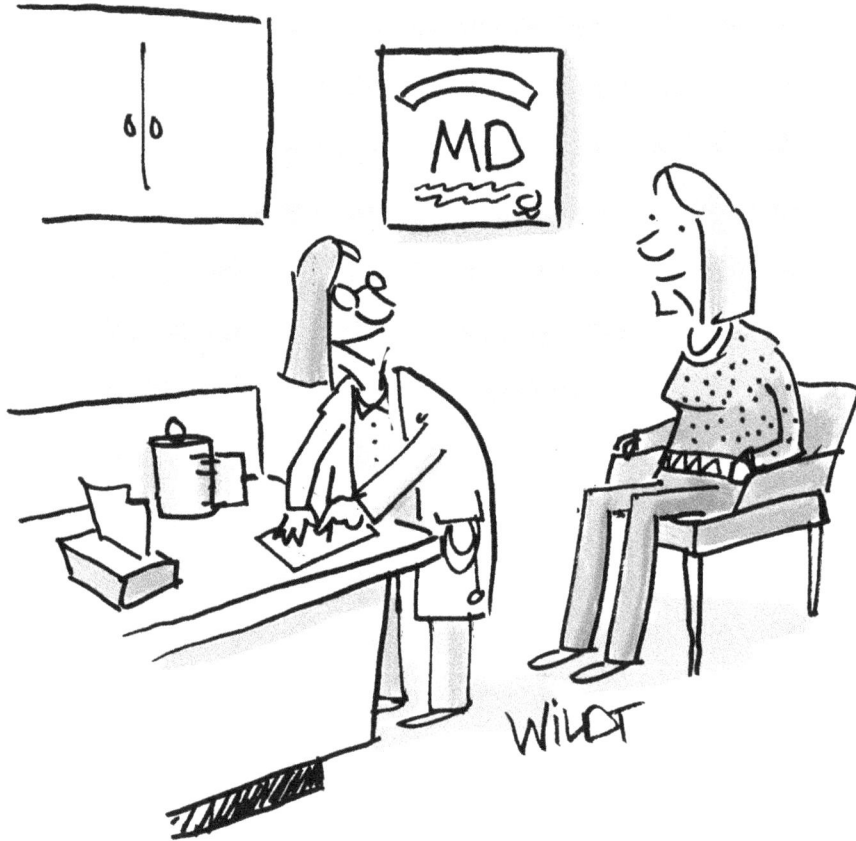

"I'm prescribing an over-the-counter relaxer.
Your local wine merchant can fill it for you."

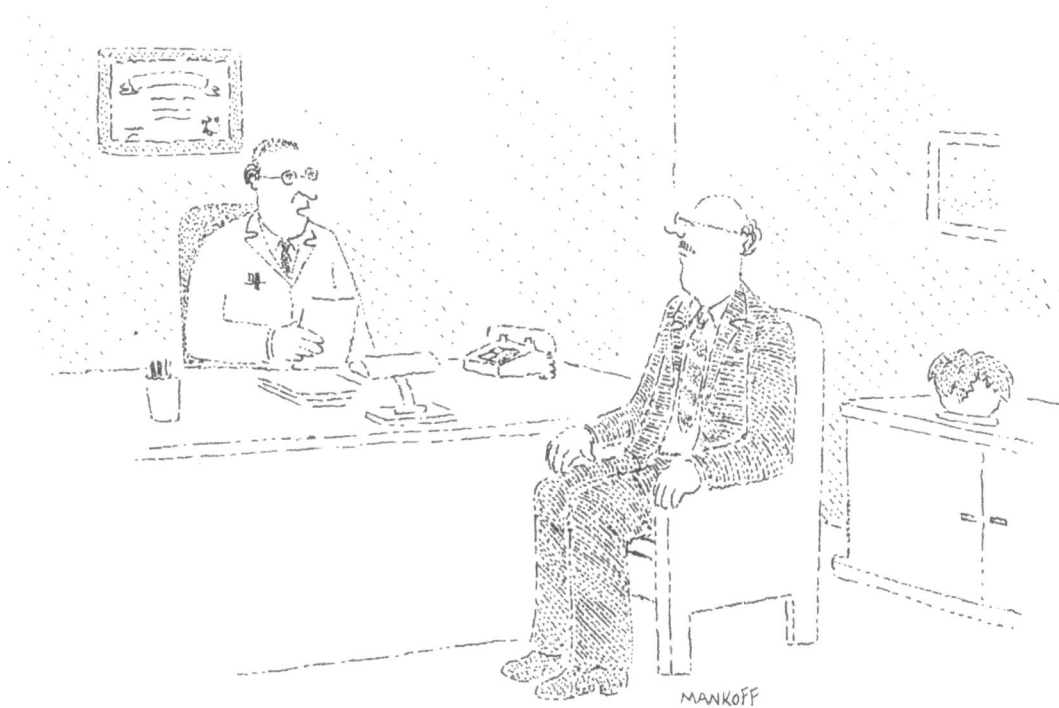

"Well, Phil, after years of vague complaints and imaginary ailments, we finally have something to work with."

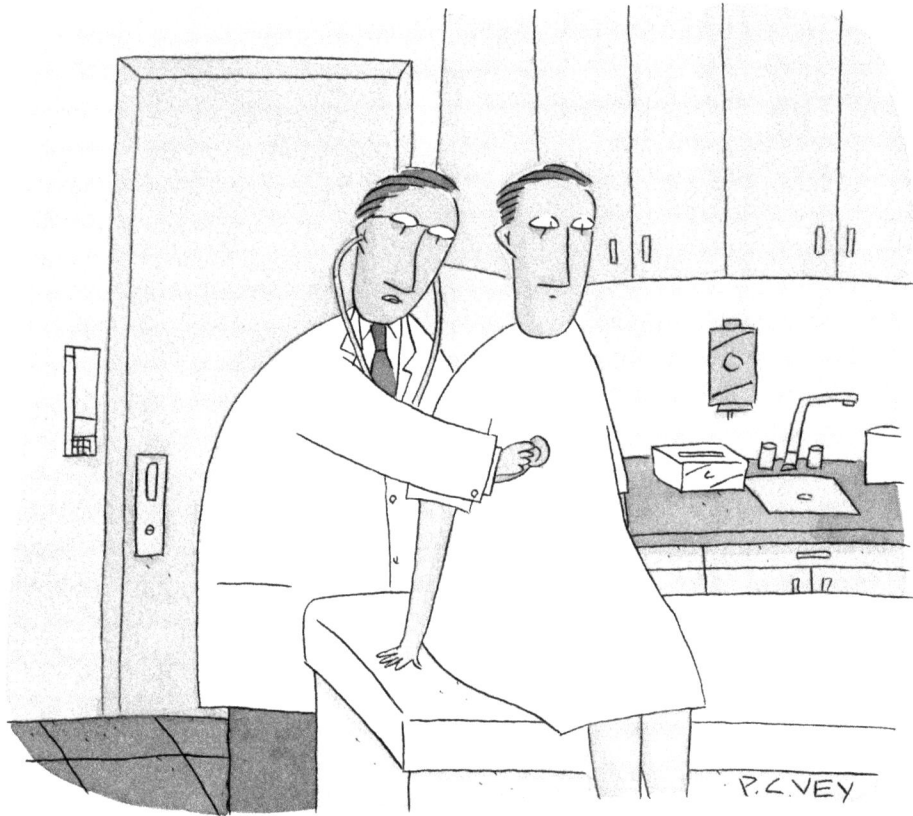

"Okay, now breathe another sigh of relief."

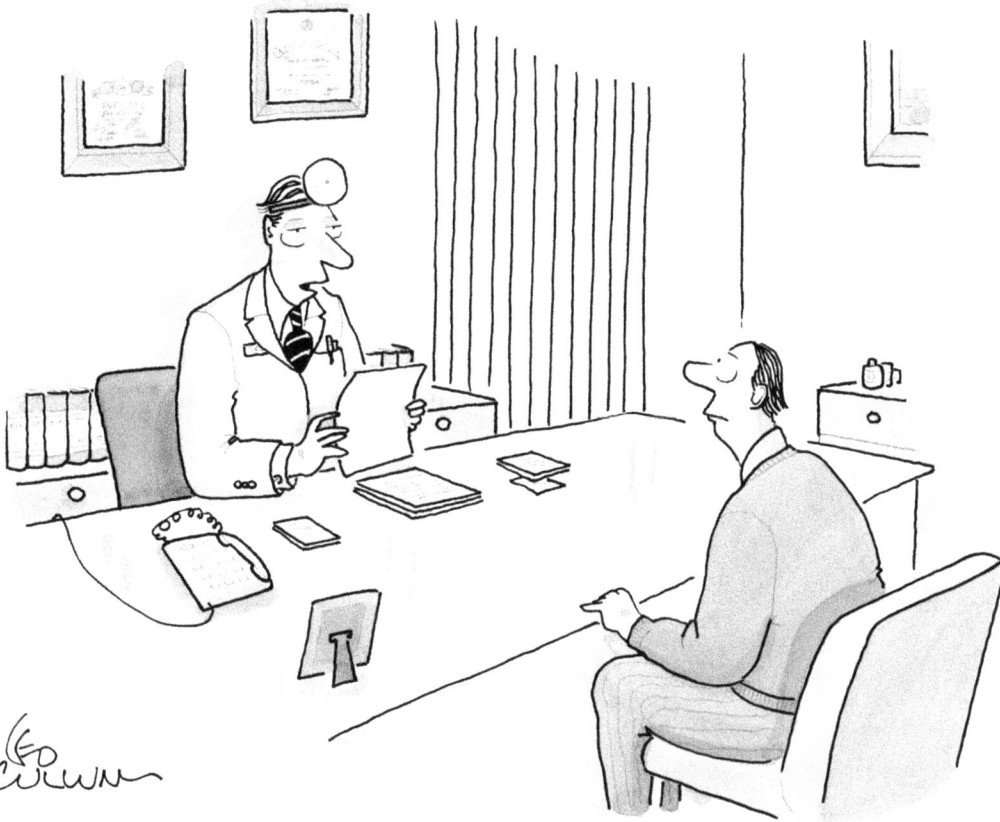

"You're fifty-seven years old. I'd like to get that down a bit."

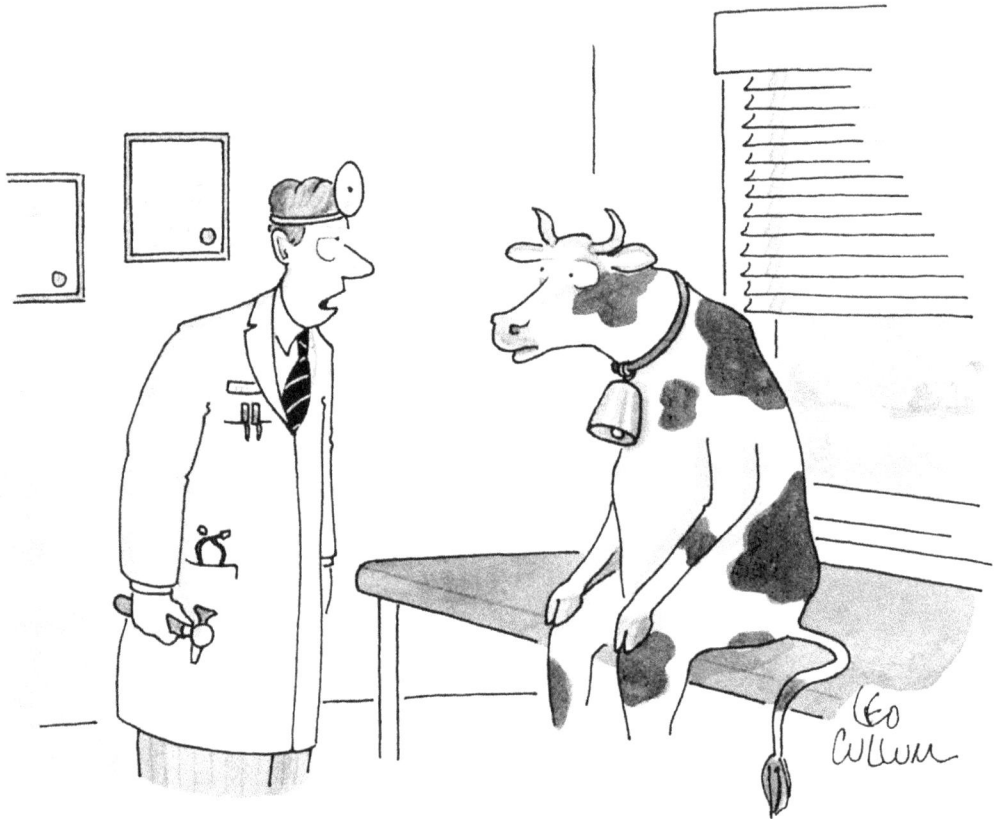

"The ringing in your ears—I think I can help."

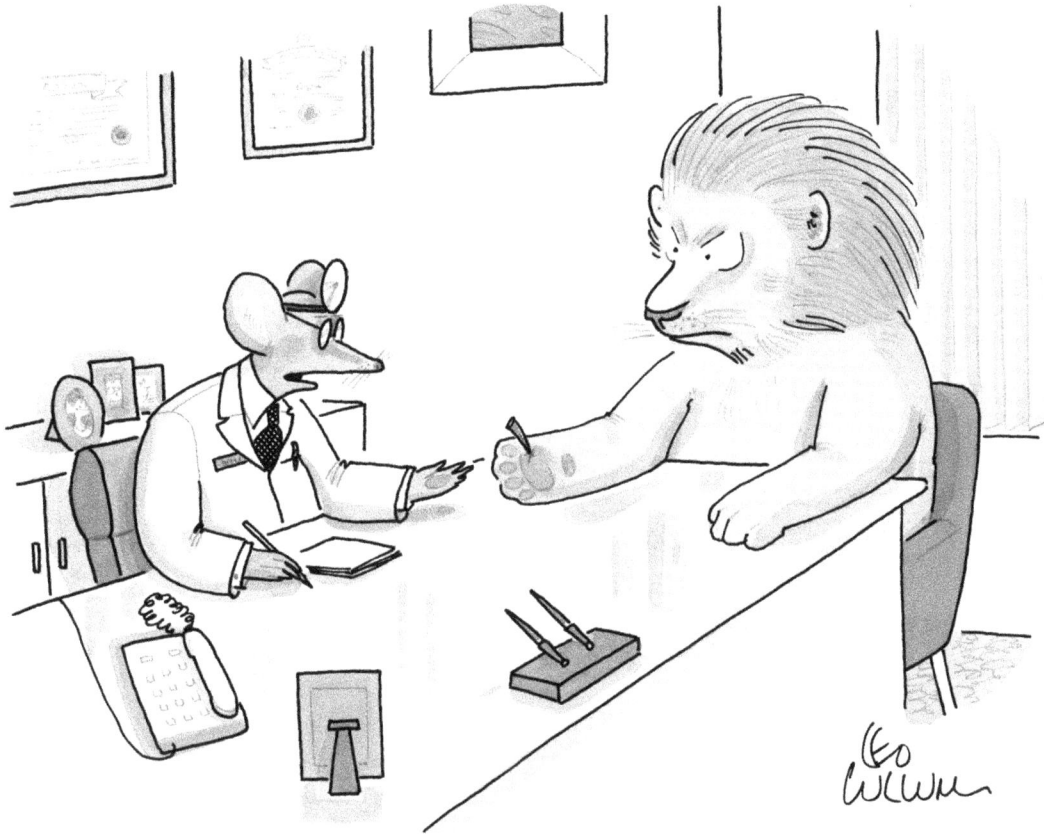

"It is thornlike in appearance, but I need to order a battery of tests."

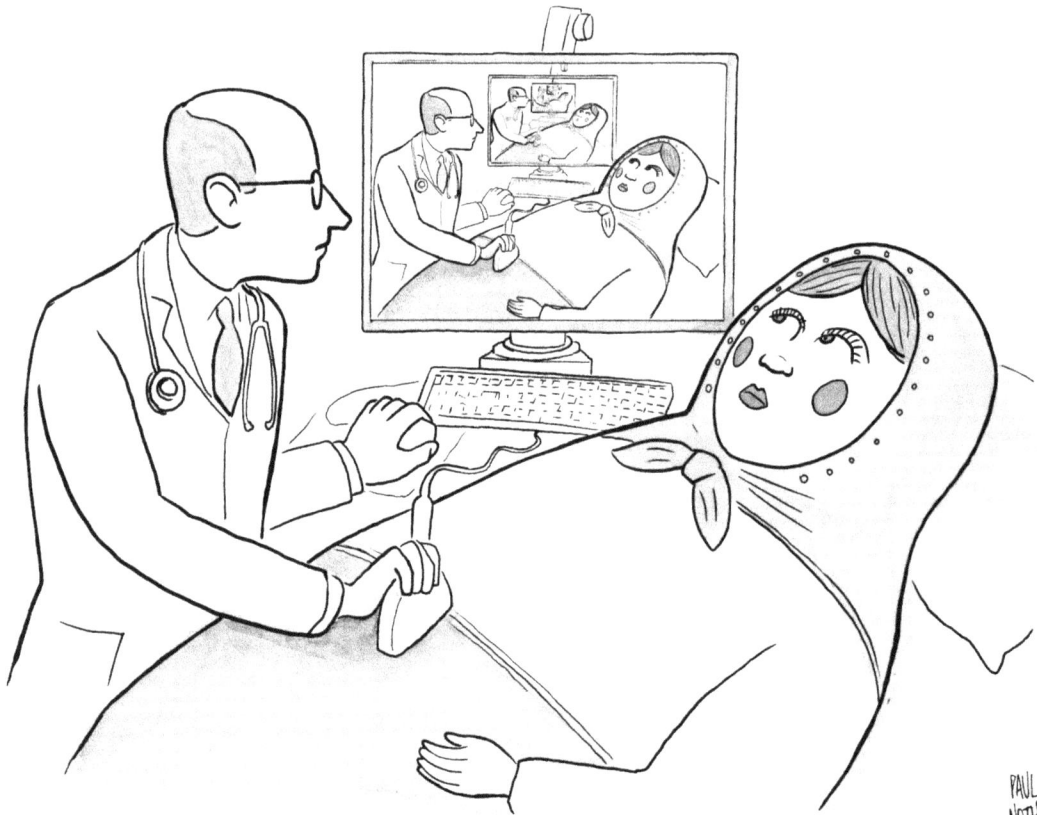

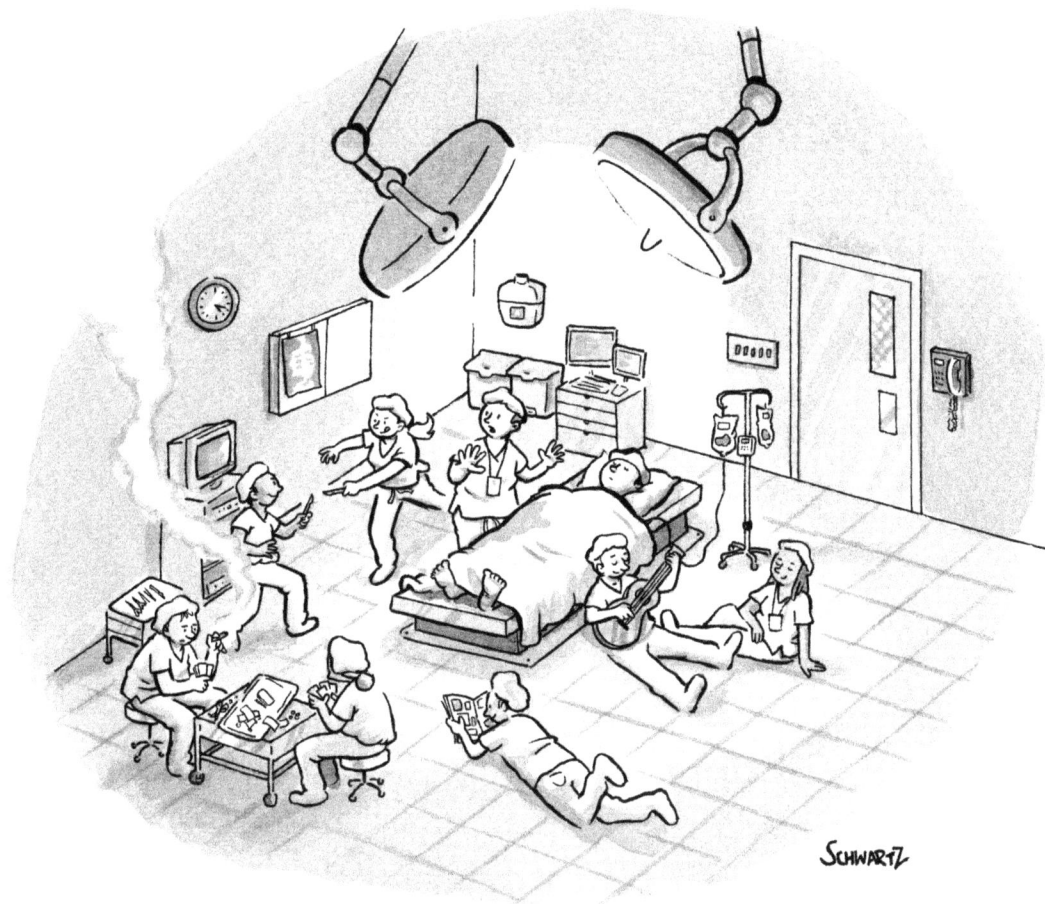

"He's waking up! Places, people!"

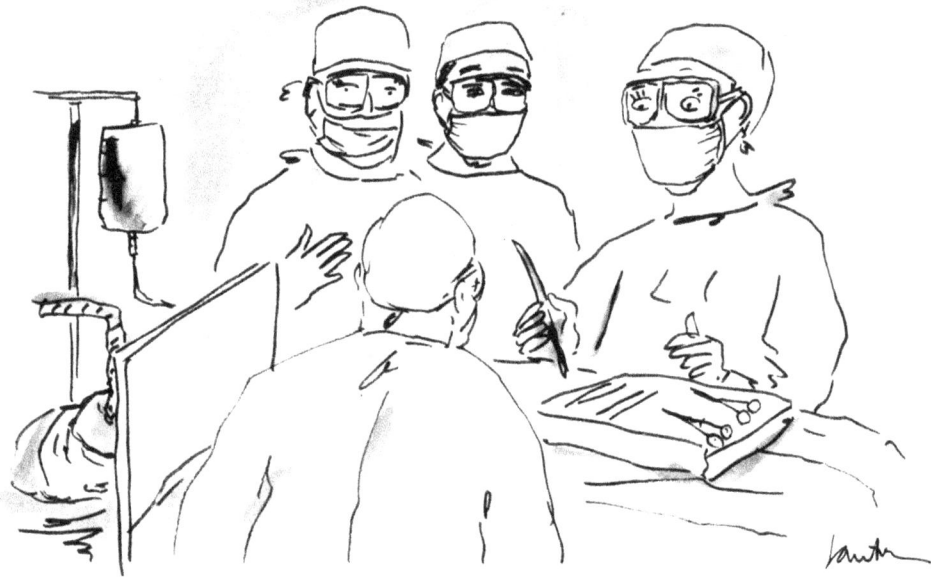

"I shouldn't have cut him open, he's not ripe."

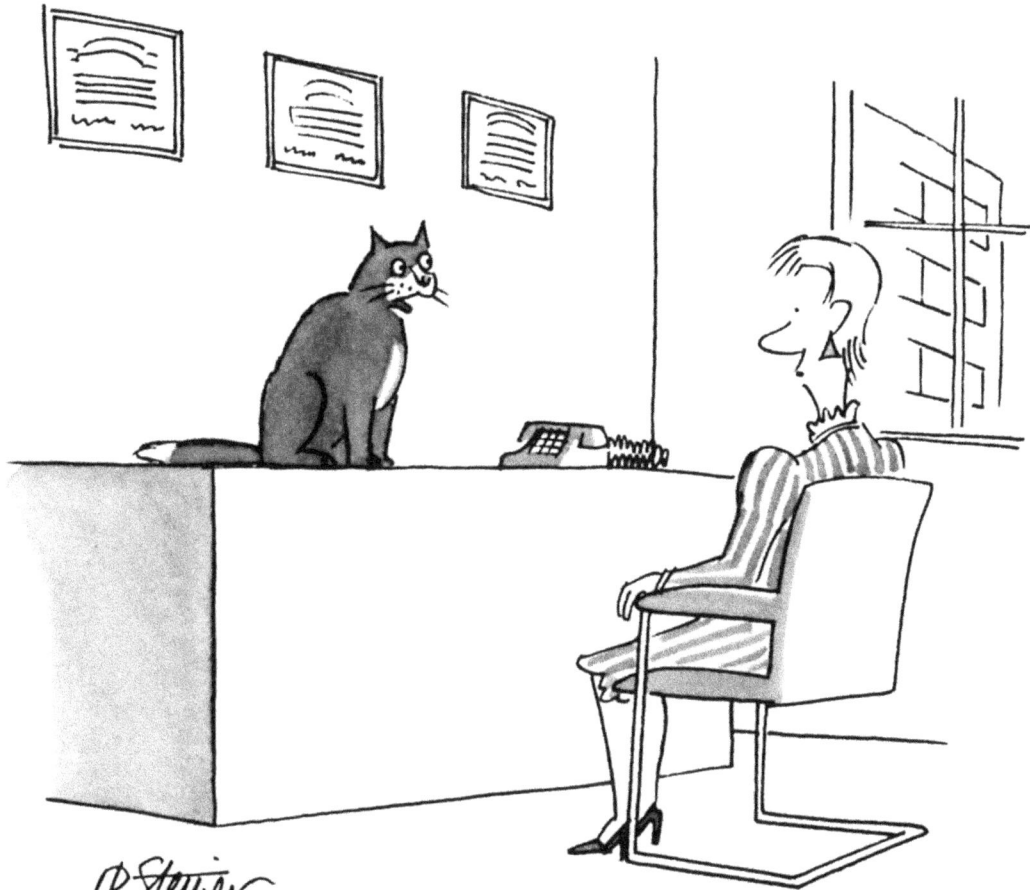

"I'd like you to have a CAT scan."

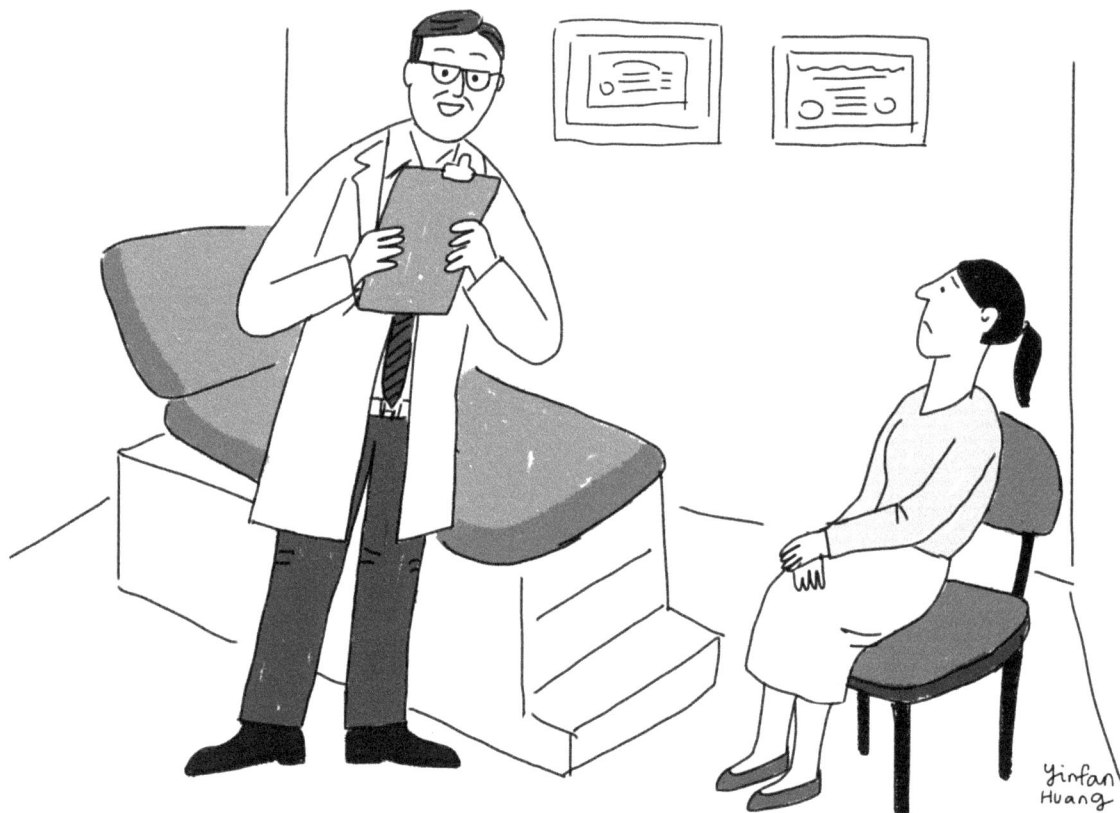

"Today we're going to do some tests which will result to something harmless but messes up your mental health."

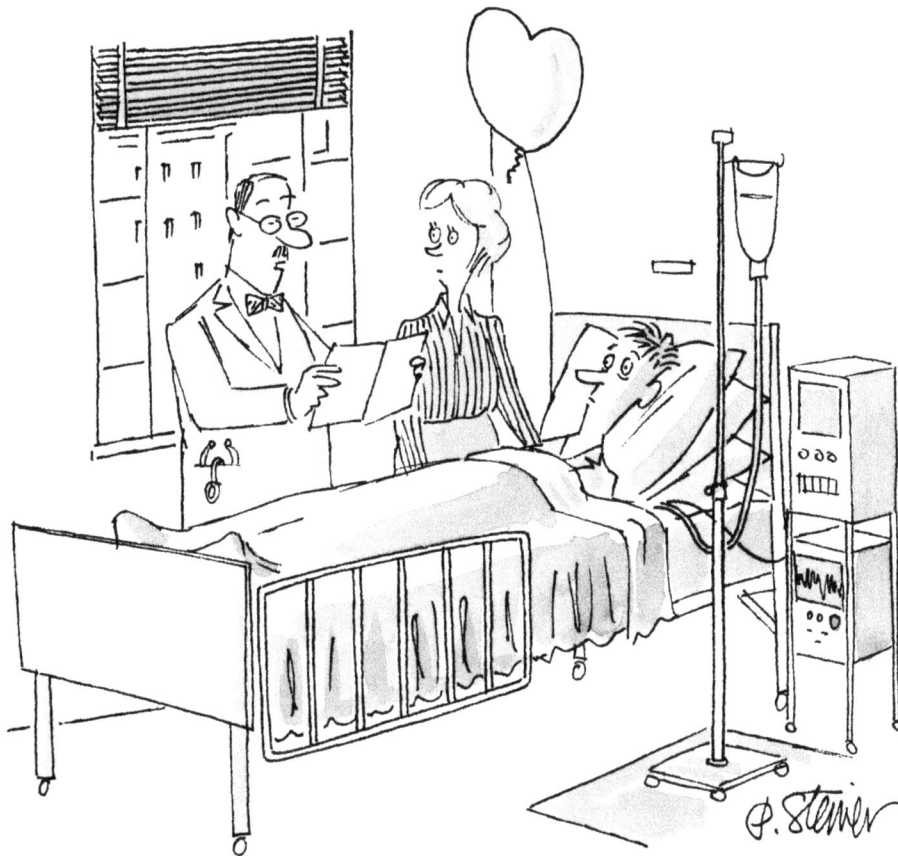

"We can give you enough medication to alleviate
the pain, but not enough to make it fun."

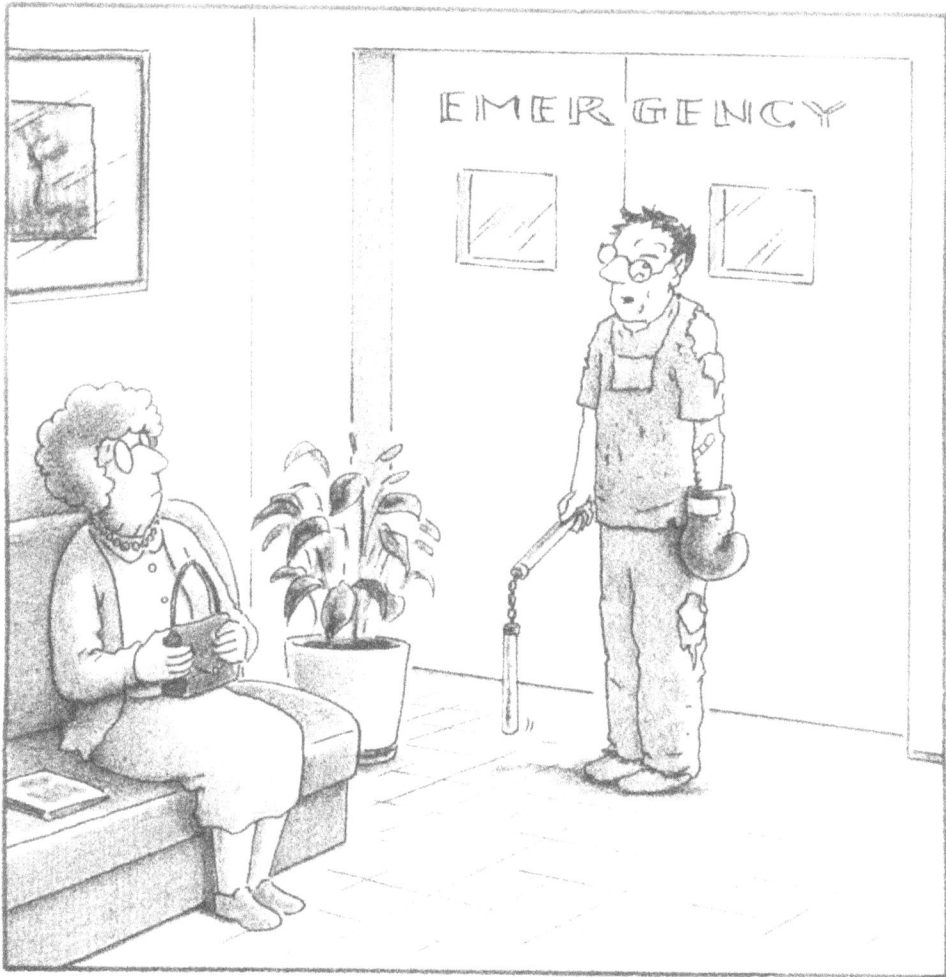

"He fought like hell."

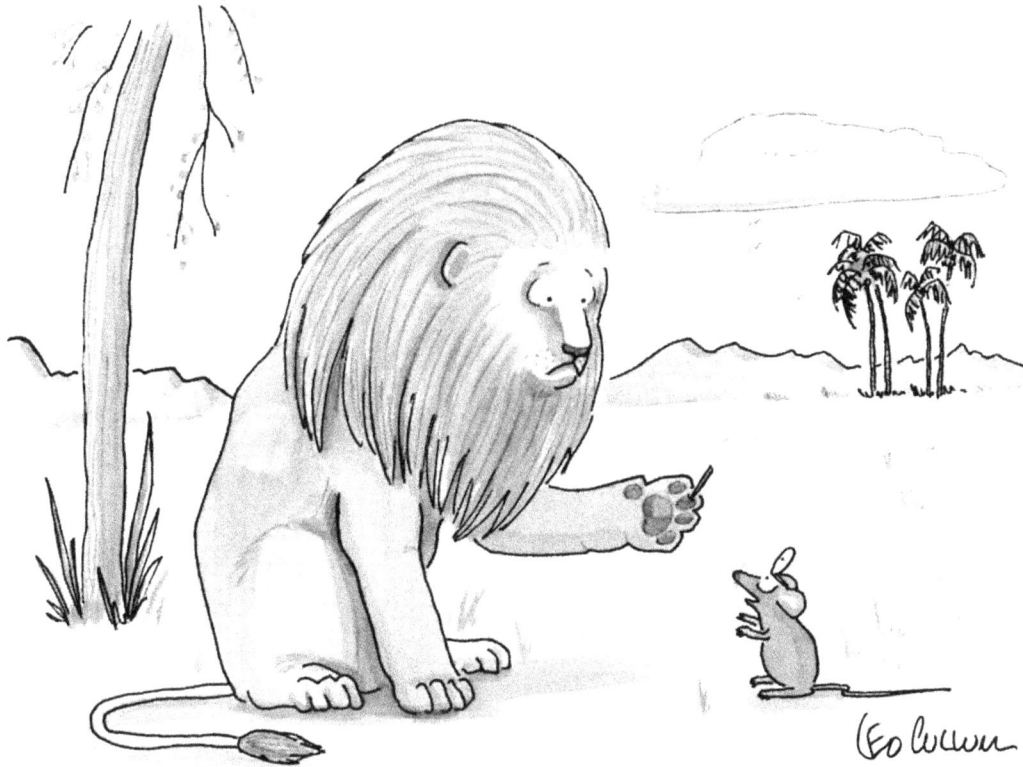

"I'd like to help you, but you're in a different H.M.O."

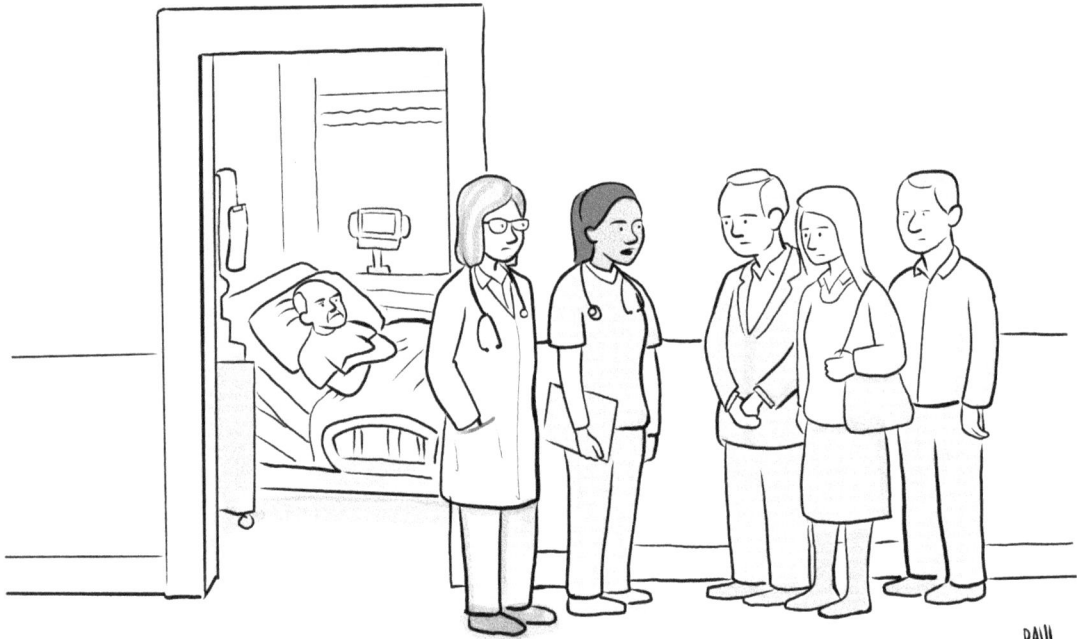

"We're doing everything we can to make him comfortable, short of dressing up as male doctors."

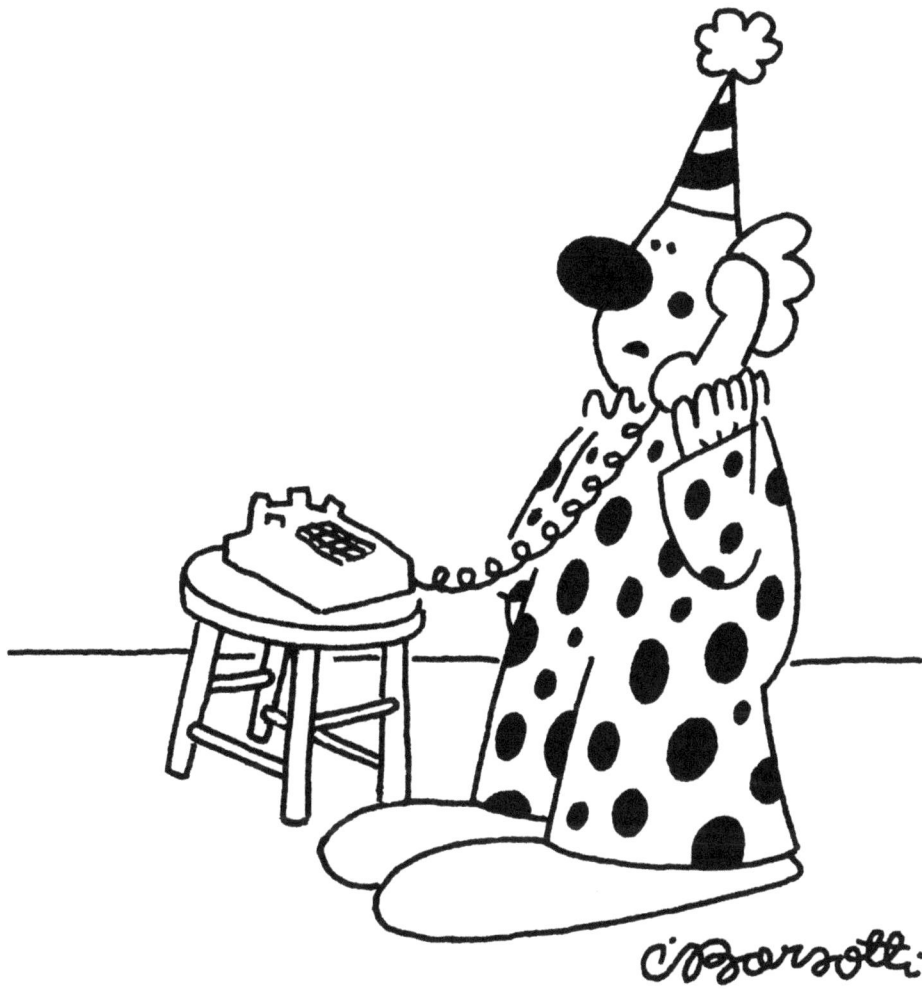

"What's the next best medicine?"

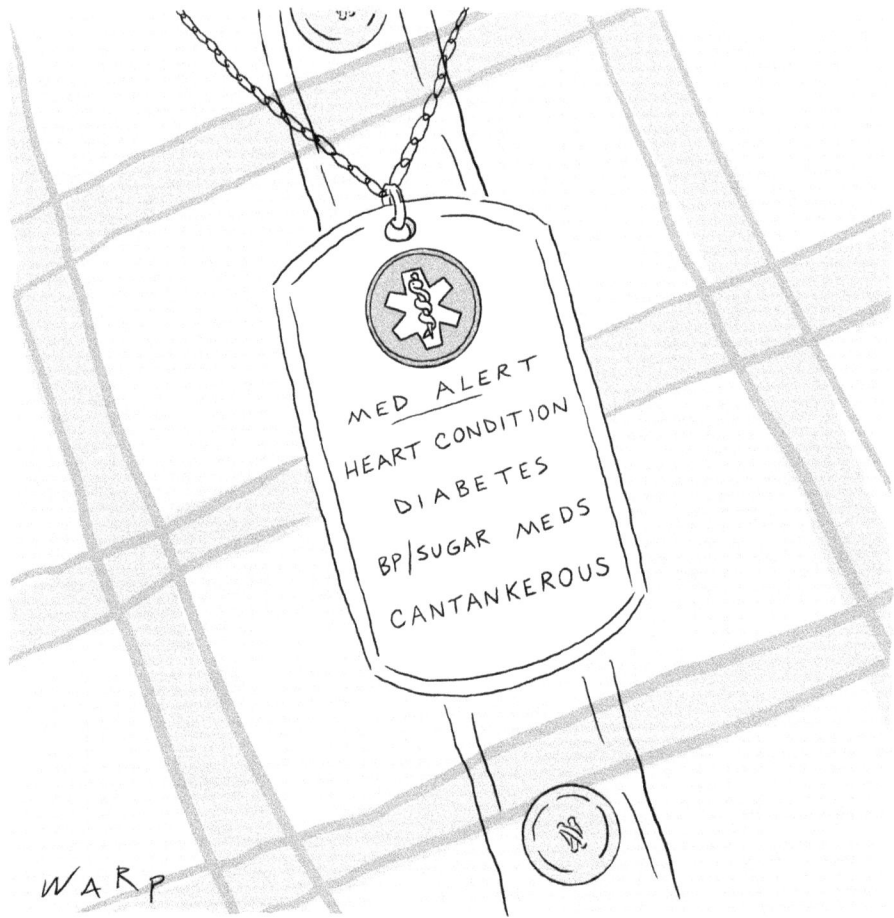

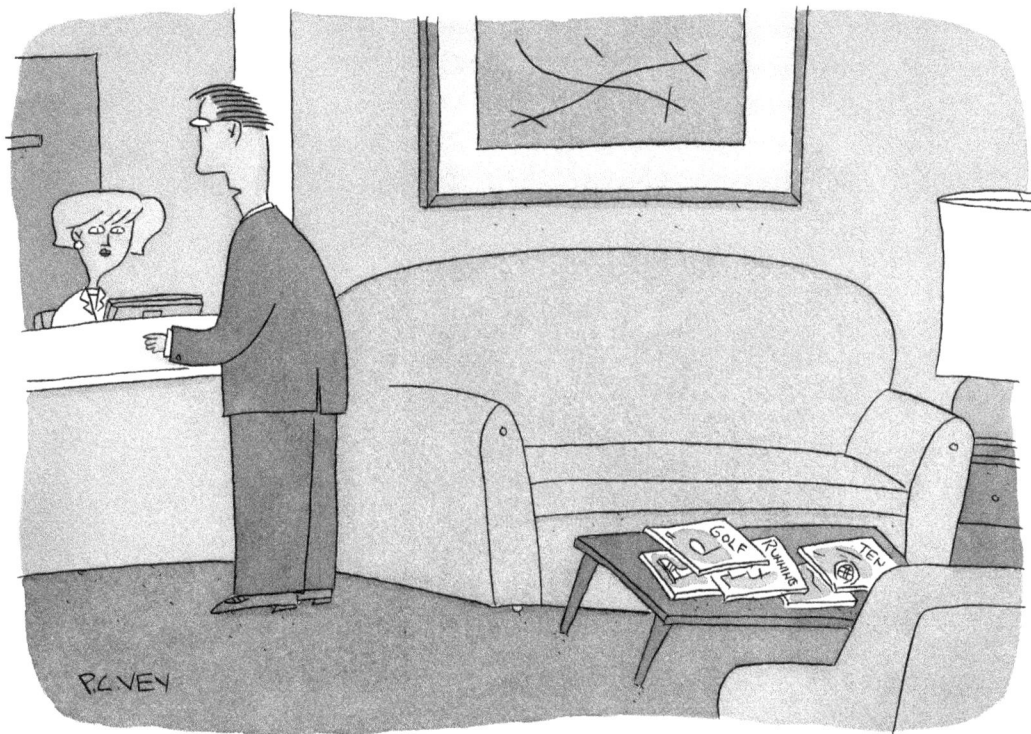

"Do you have any reading material that doesn't mock the sedentary life?"

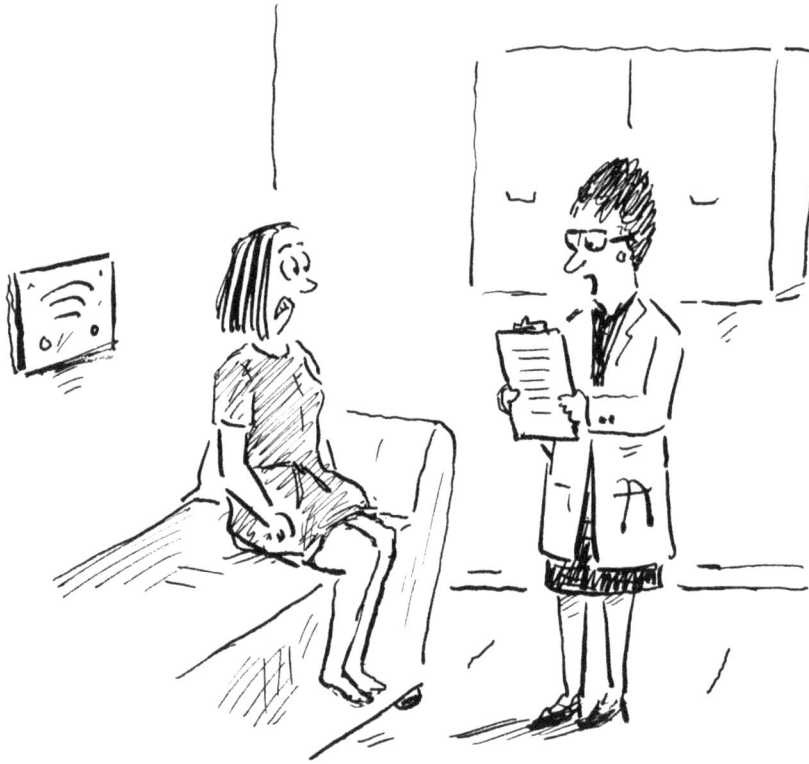

SIPRESS

"I'm going to ask you a series of scary questions. When I'm done,
let's see if you can guess why I'm asking them."

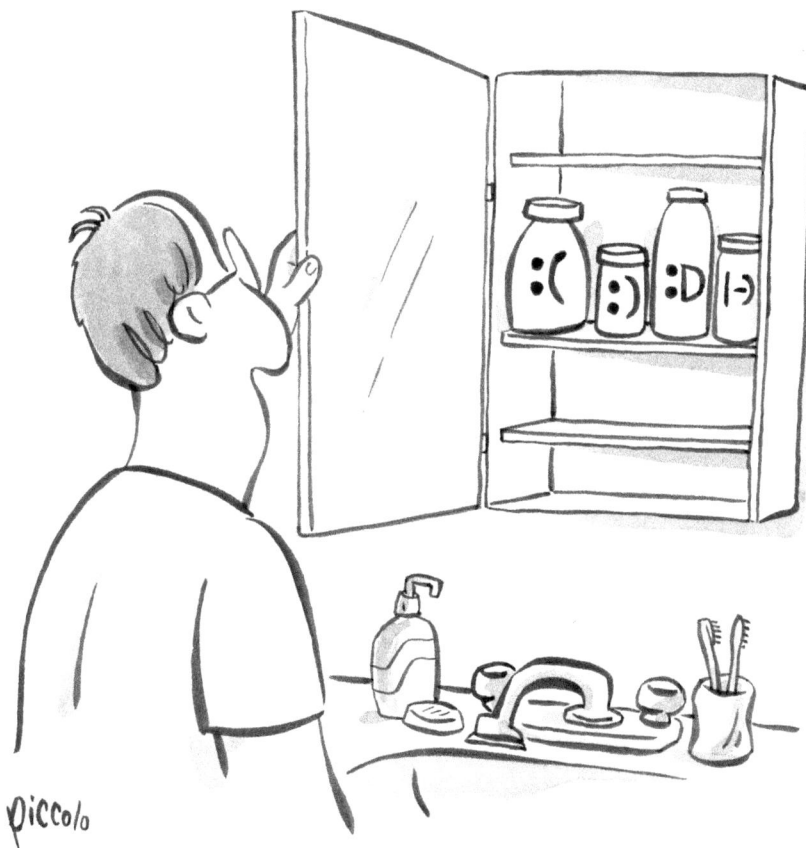

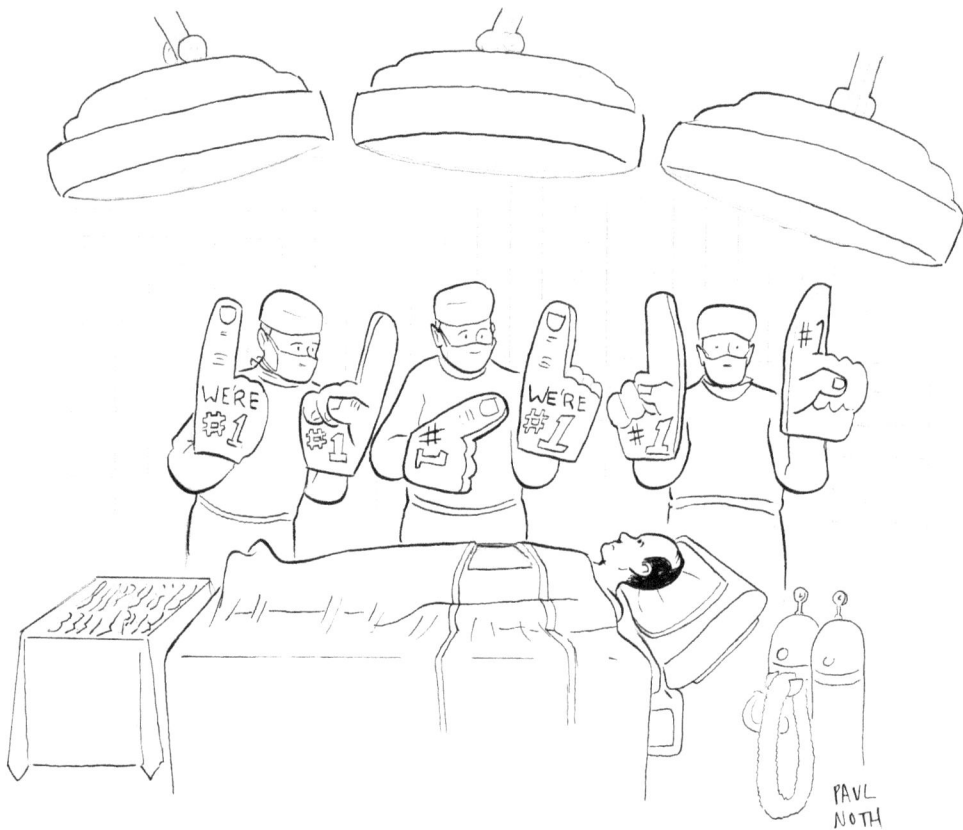

"We lose a little dexterity, but we gain a lot of confidence."

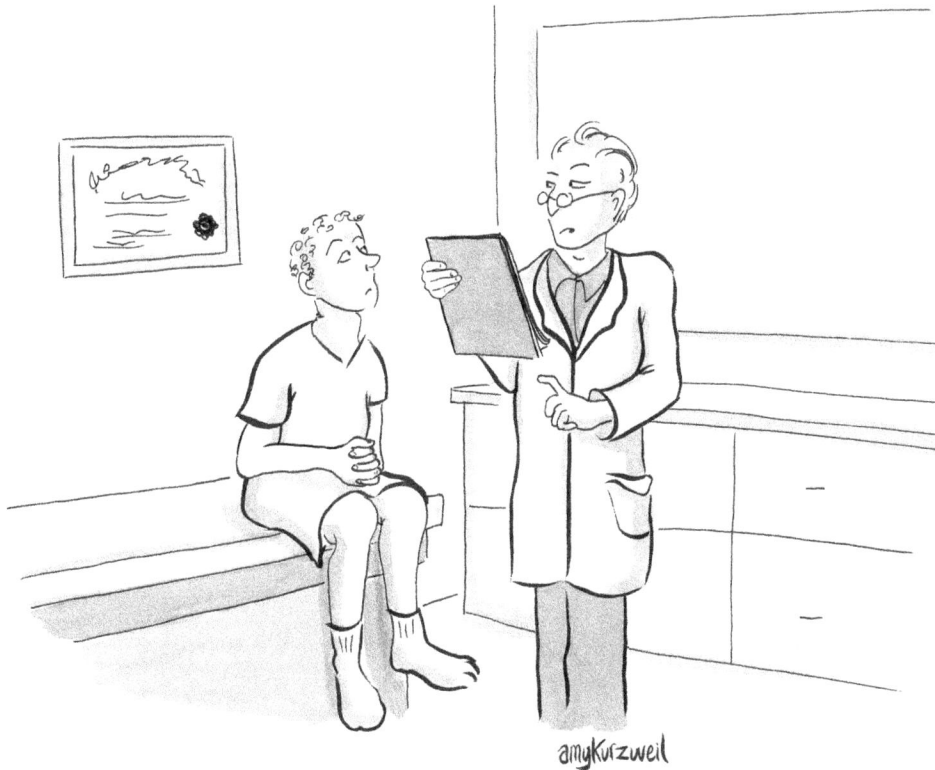

"*Your tests look normal, but that's what the disease wants us to think.*"

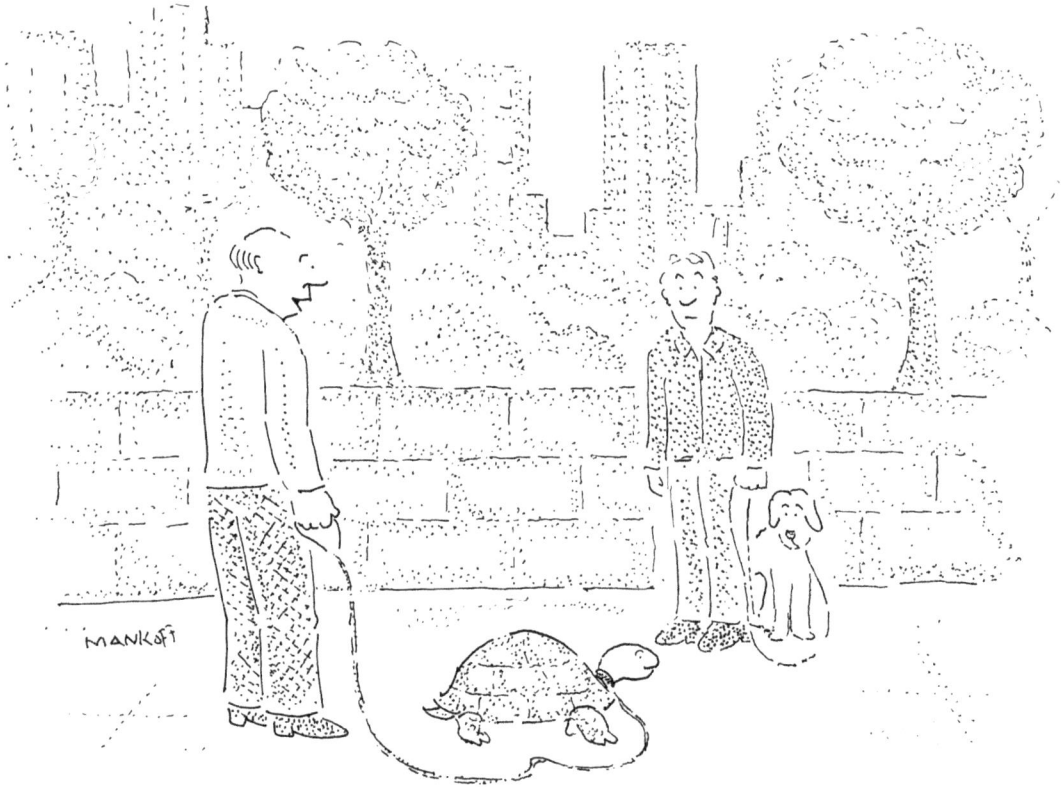

"*My doctor told me to take it easy.*"

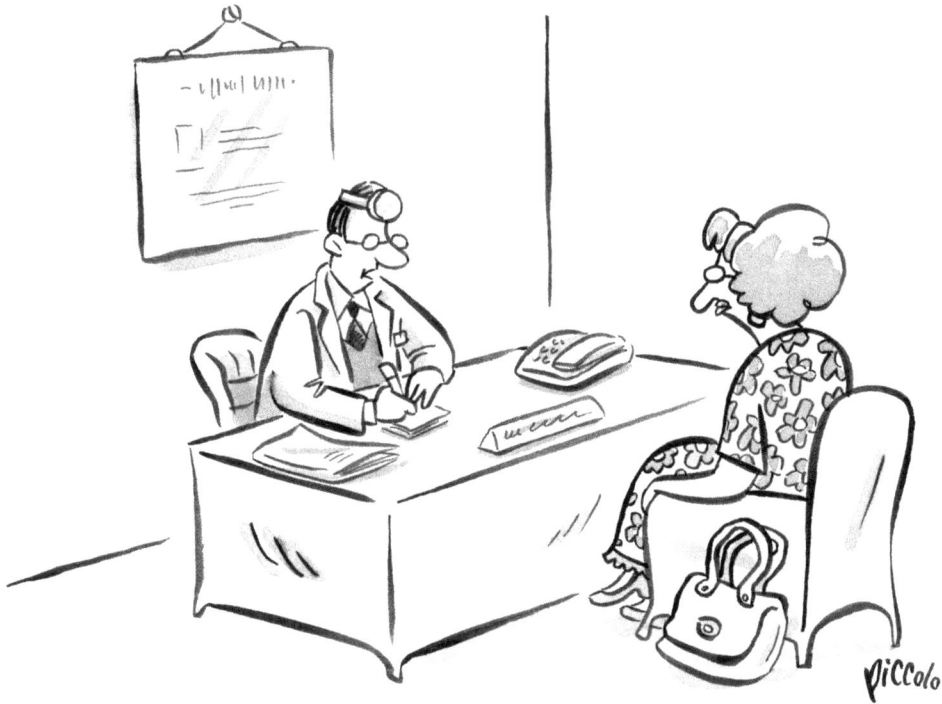

"I'm going to prescribe medical marijuana
and sour cream & onion tortilla chips."

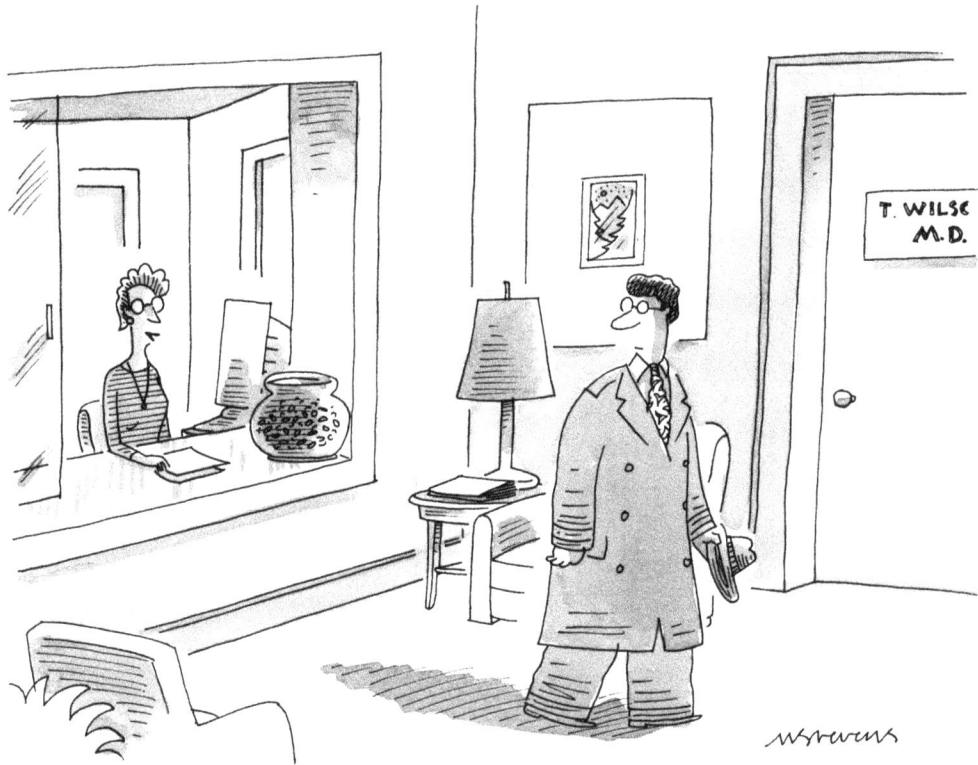

"Don't forget to take a handful of our complimentary antibiotics on your way out."

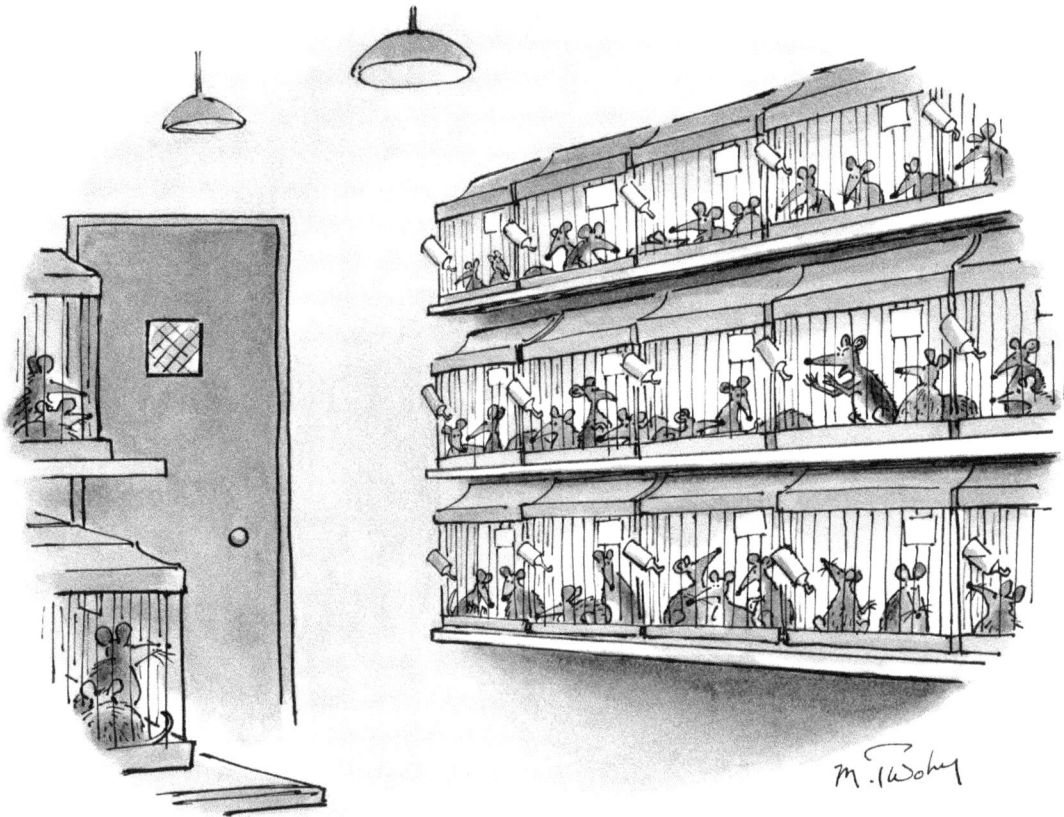

"When Dr. Henderson comes in, everybody play dead."

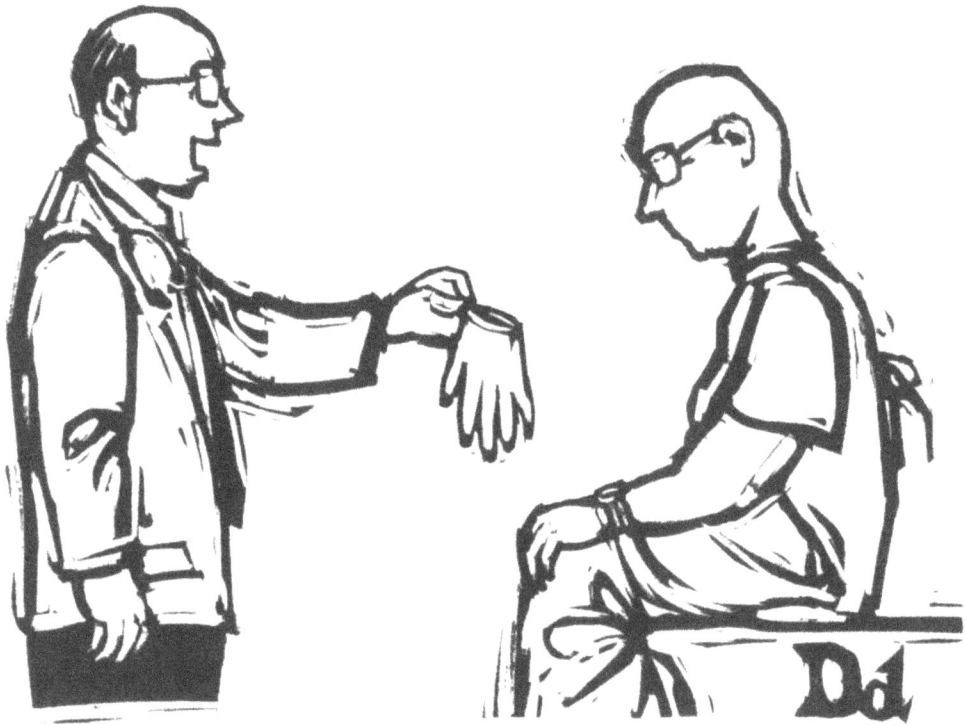

"Give a man an exam and he'll be healthy for a day;
teach a man to examine himself and he'll be healthy for a lifetime."

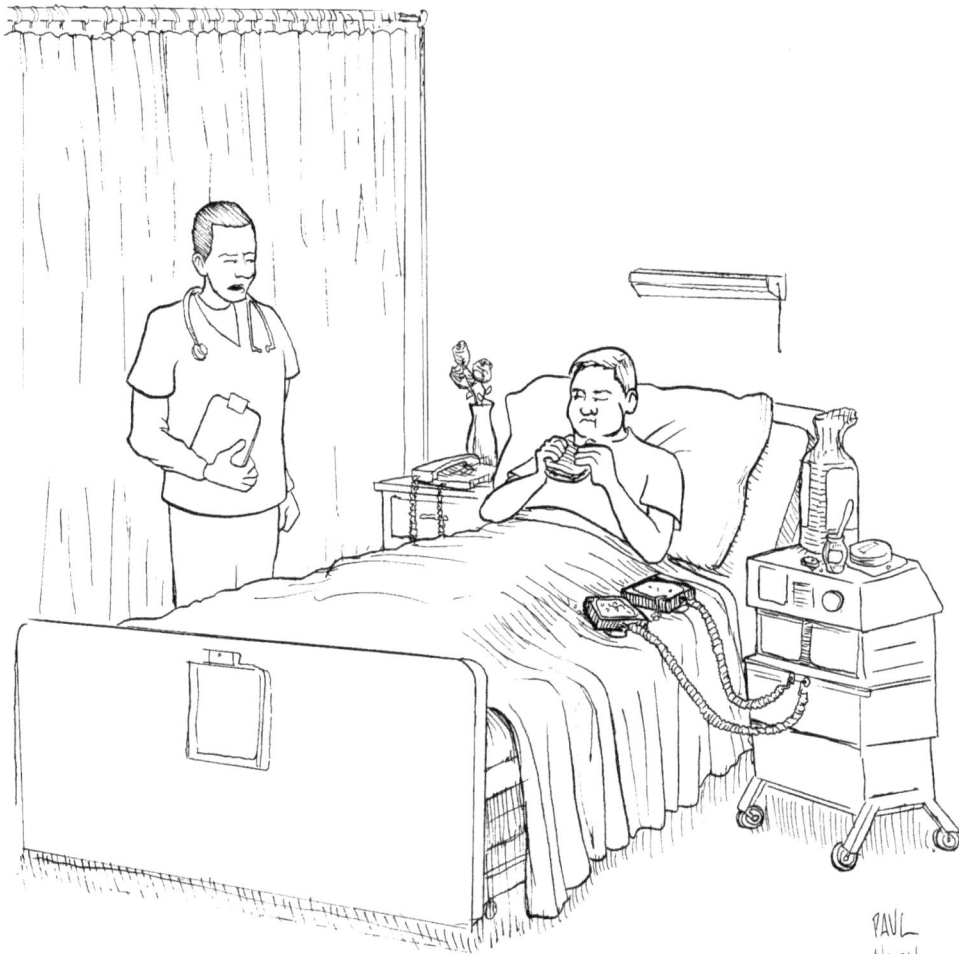

"The defibrillator's not for pressing panini."

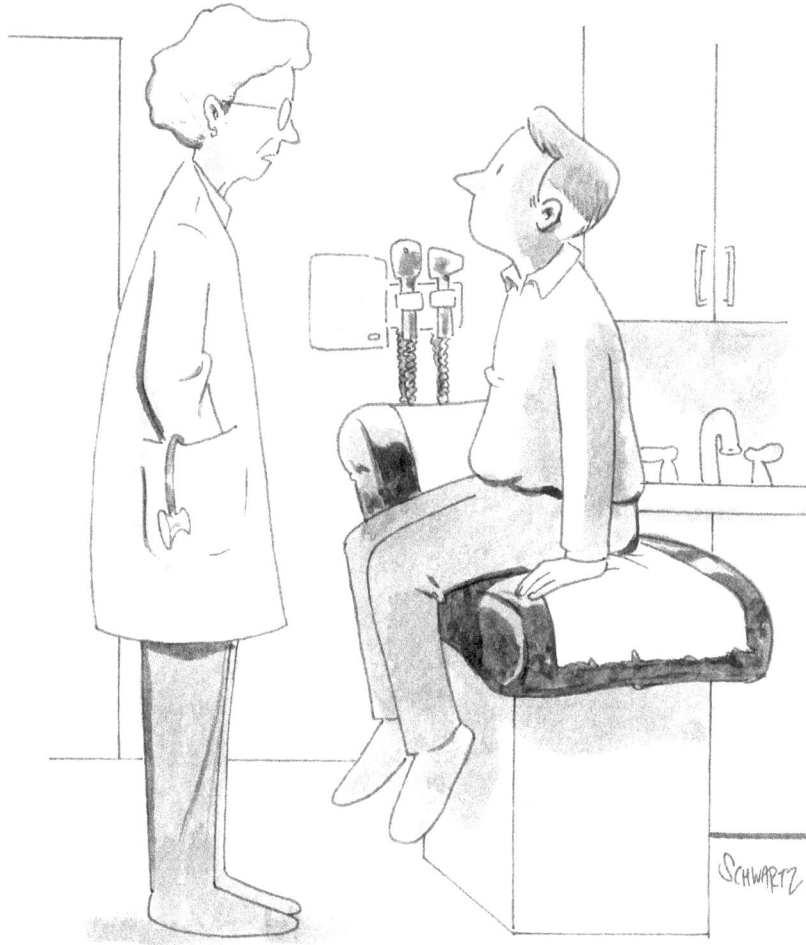

"We can't cure it, but with enough social pressure, we can get it cancelled."

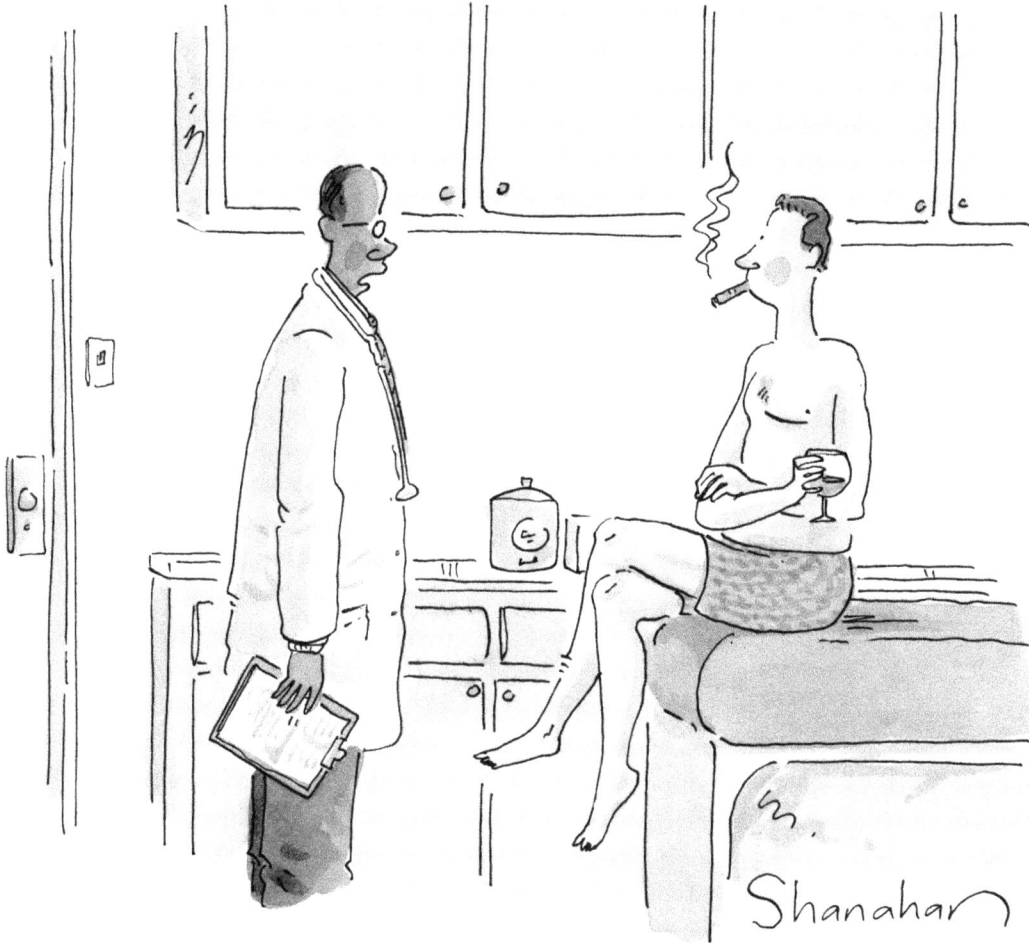

"You should relax less."

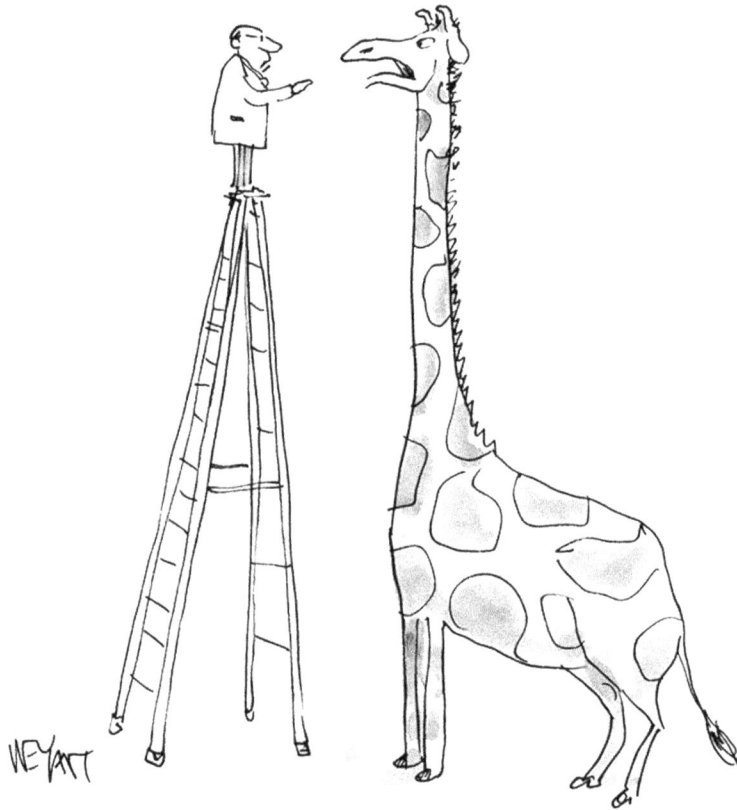

"Why do you always assume it's a sore throat?"

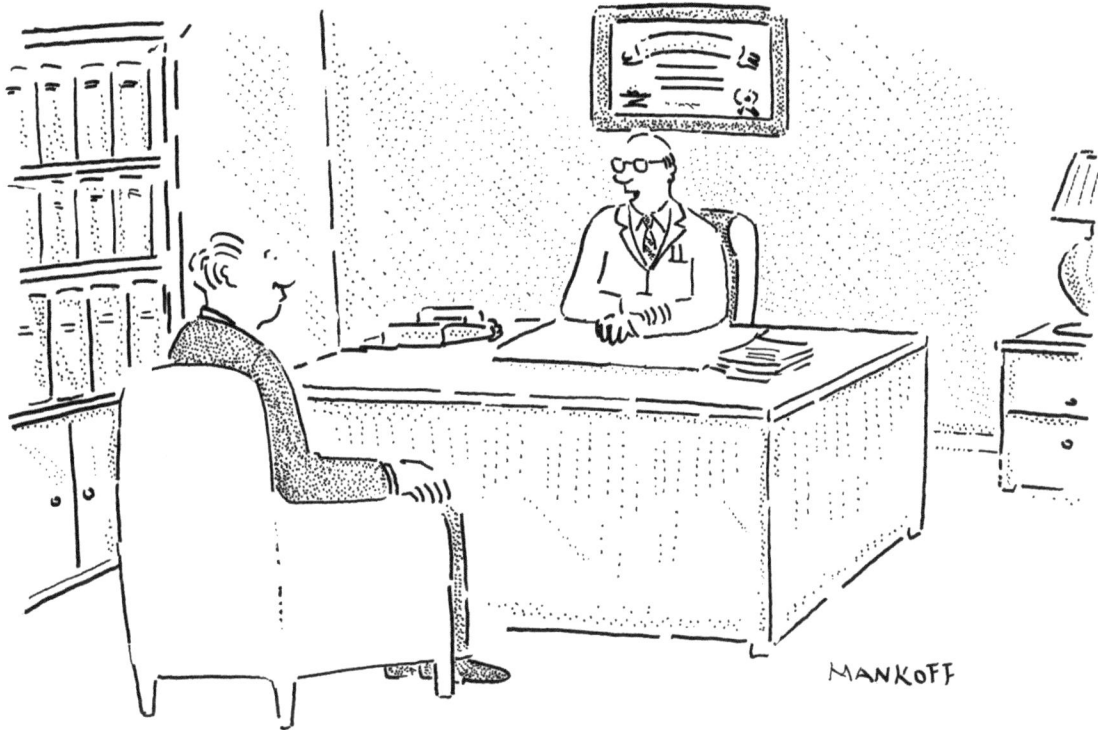

"Well, yes, it's a routine procedure – if you routinely have someone slice open your body with sharp instruments and then fiddle with your insides."

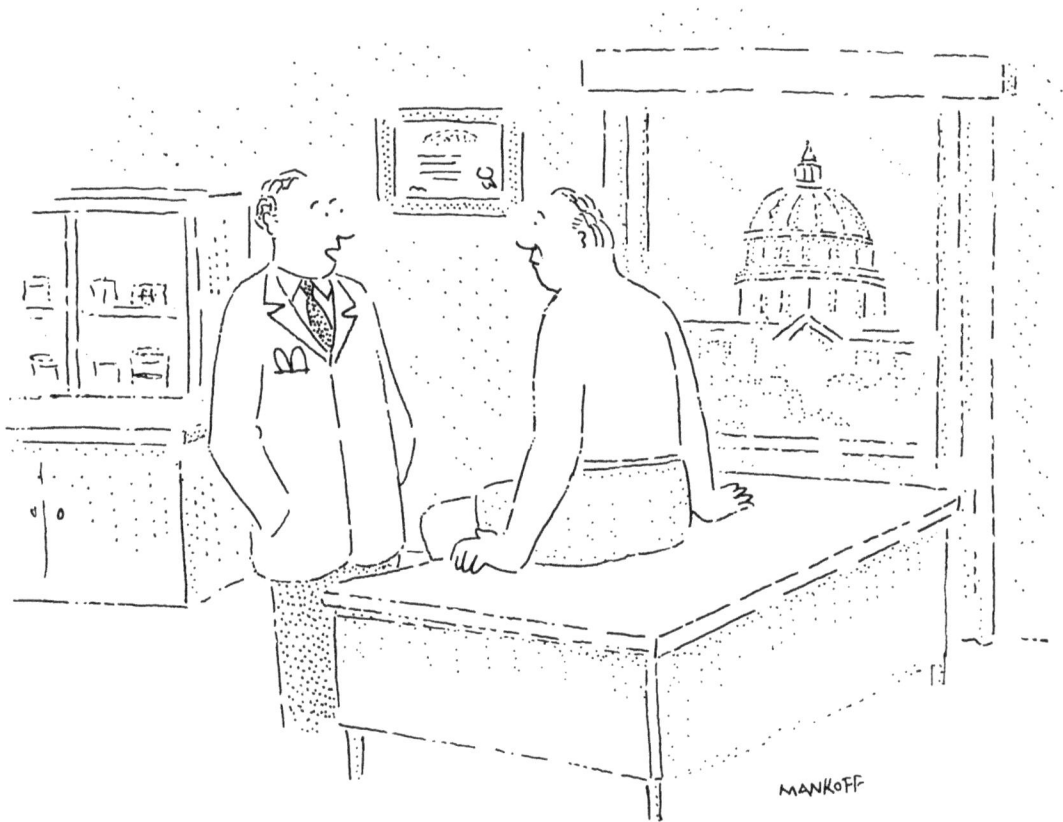

"Bad news—that fire in your belly is an ulcer."

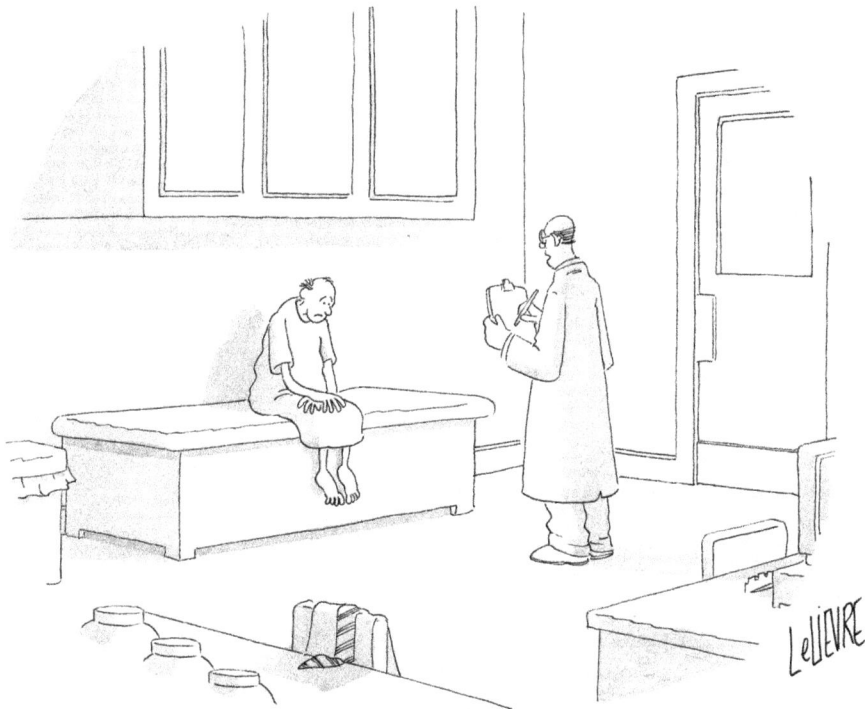

"I'm afraid you have thirty, maybe forty, years to live."

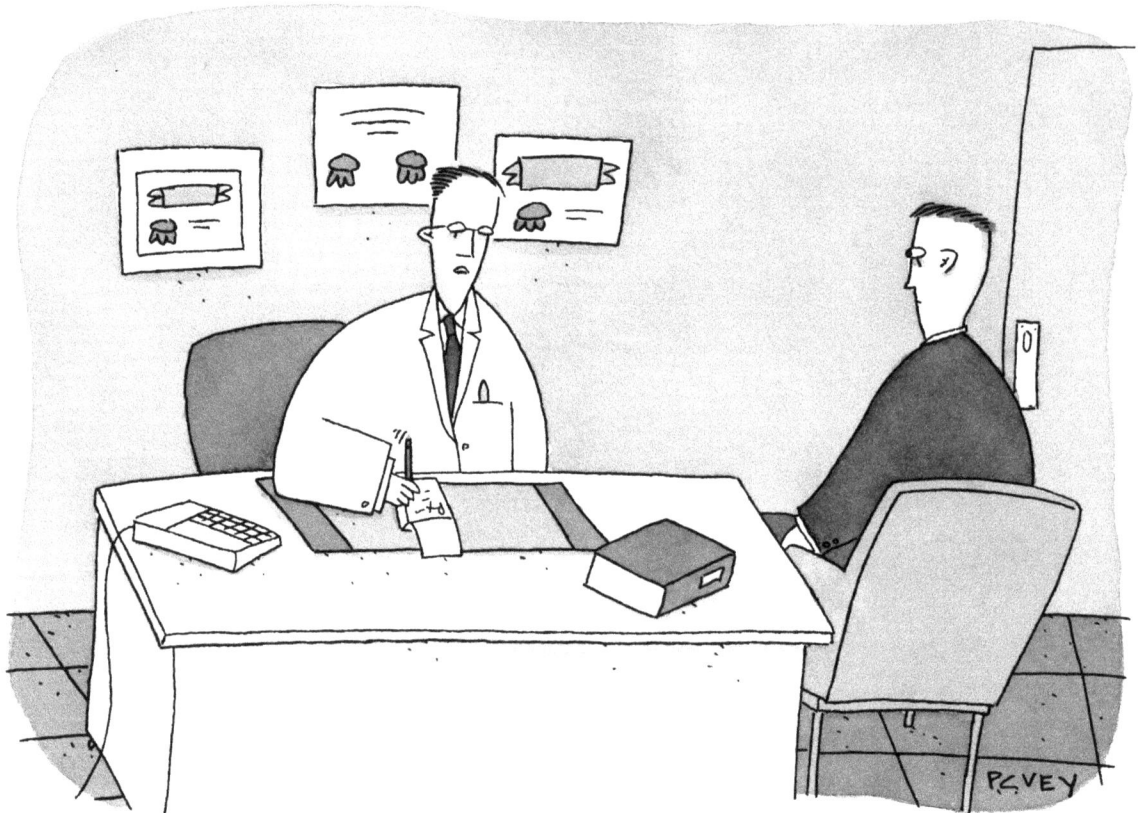

"I'm taking you off medicinal marijuana and
putting you on medicinal harder stuff."

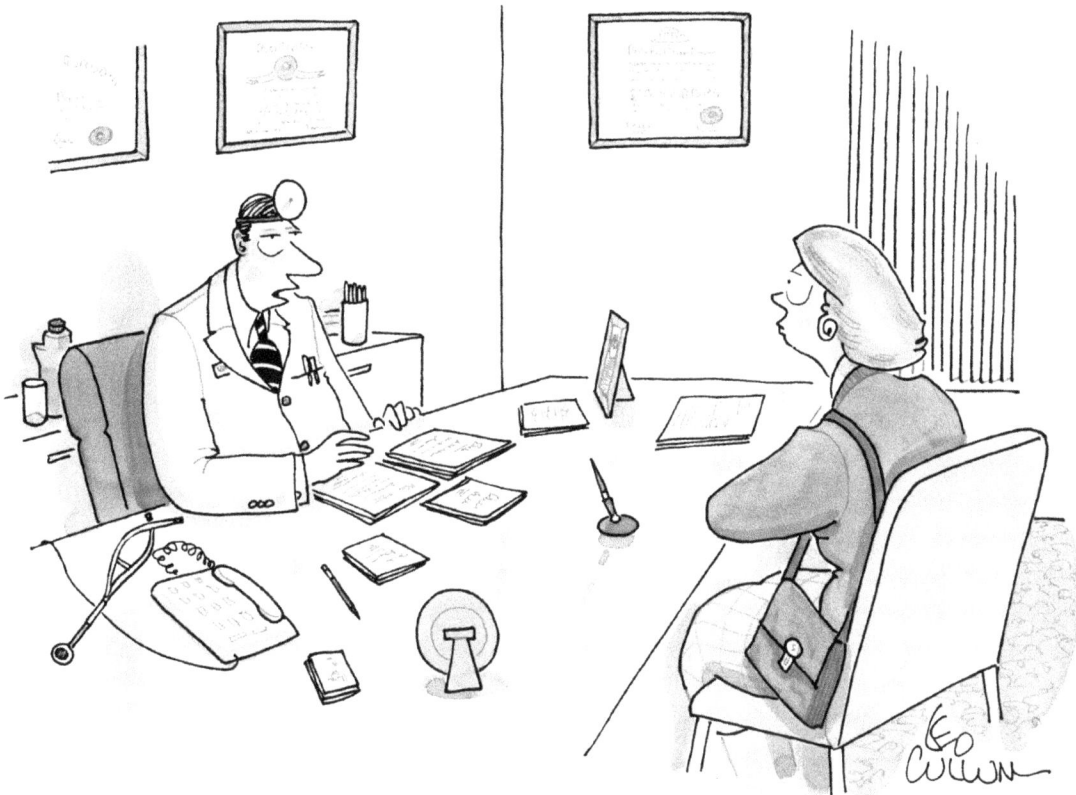

"*Have you popped all those pills I prescribed?*"

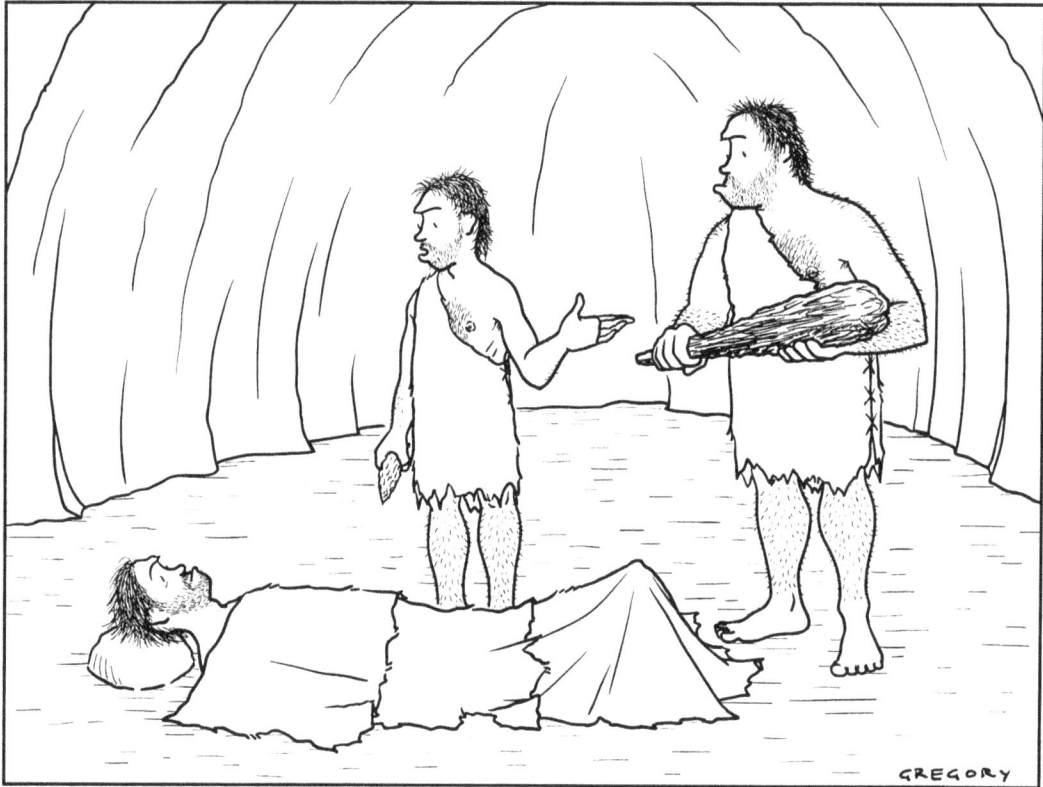

"I'll be performing the operation, and this is the anesthesiologist."

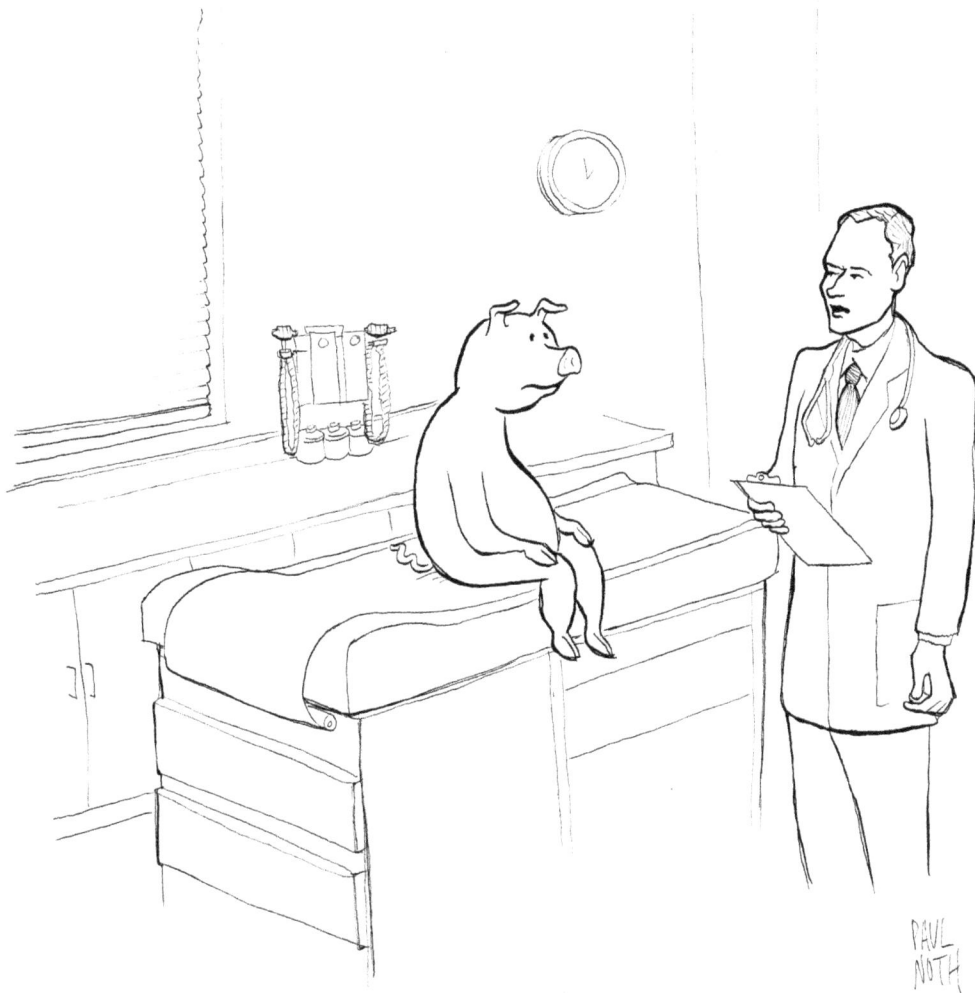

"It's your ribs. I'm afraid they're delicious."

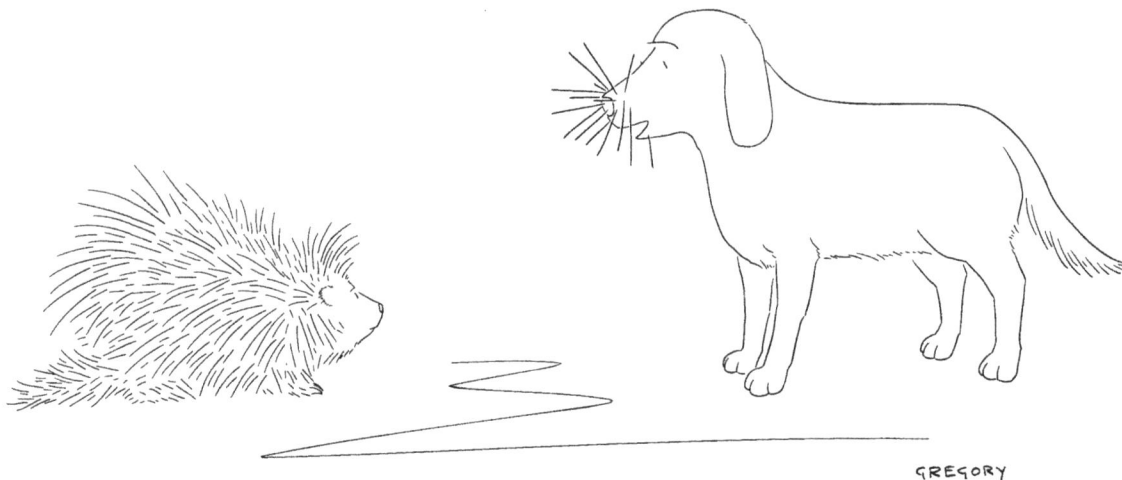

"*On the plus side, you've cured my back pain.*"

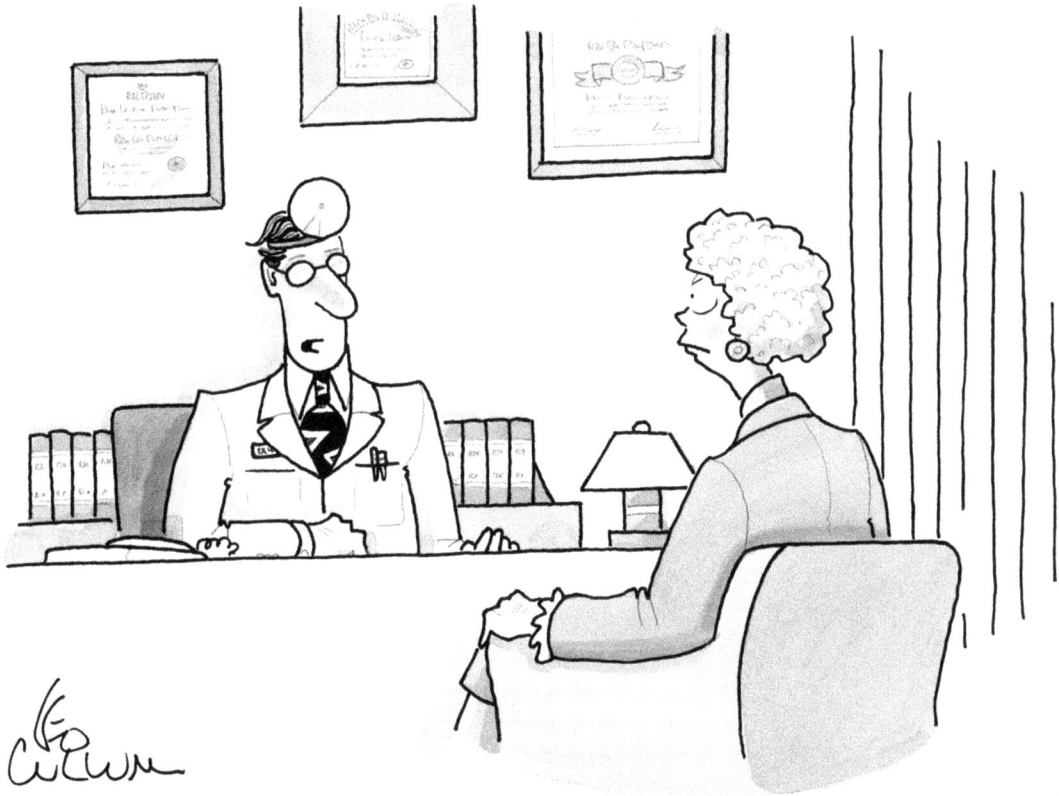

"*You may believe you've been overcharged, but, remember, you're overmedicated.*"

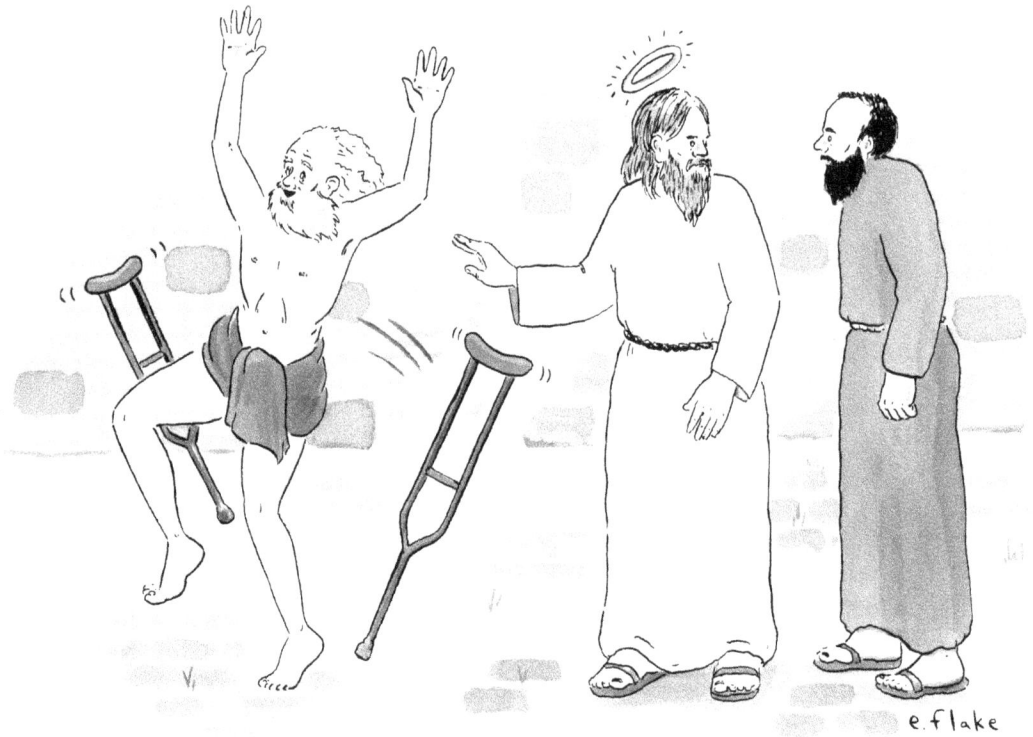

"Yeah, but good luck getting it peer-reviewed."

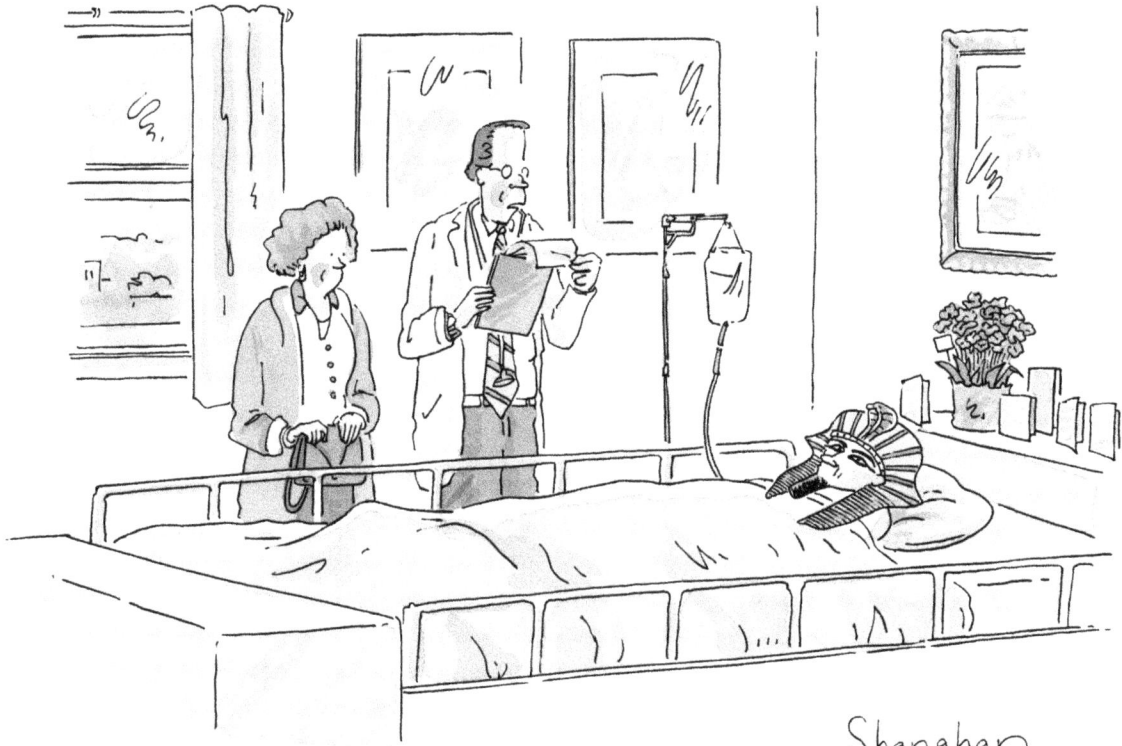

"We're pretty sure it's the West Nile Virus."

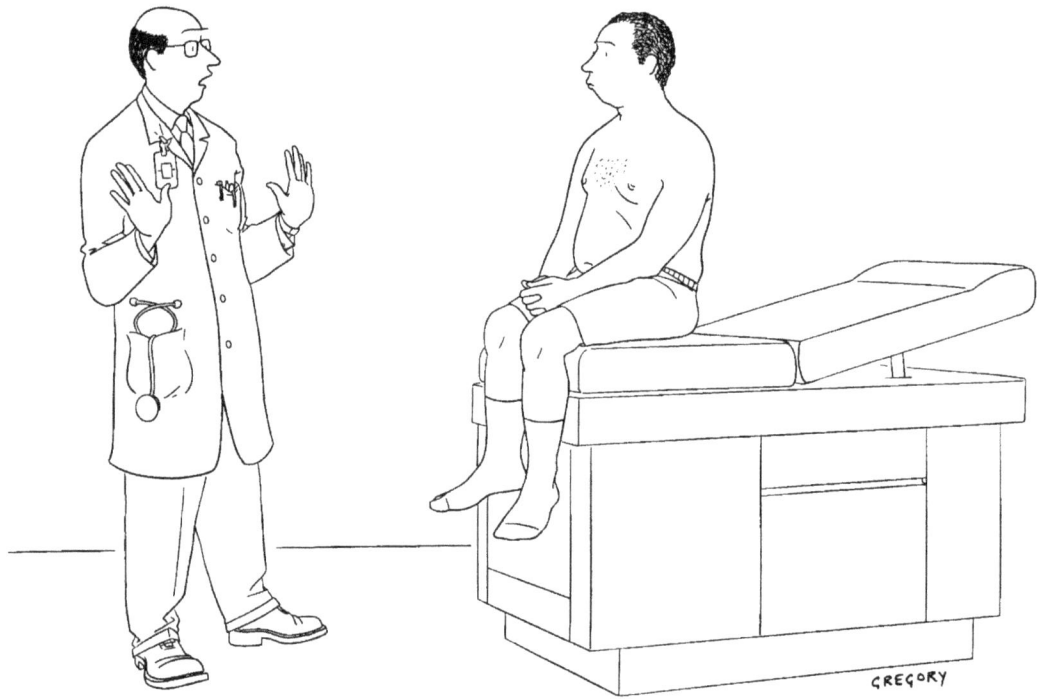

"Whoa—way too much information."

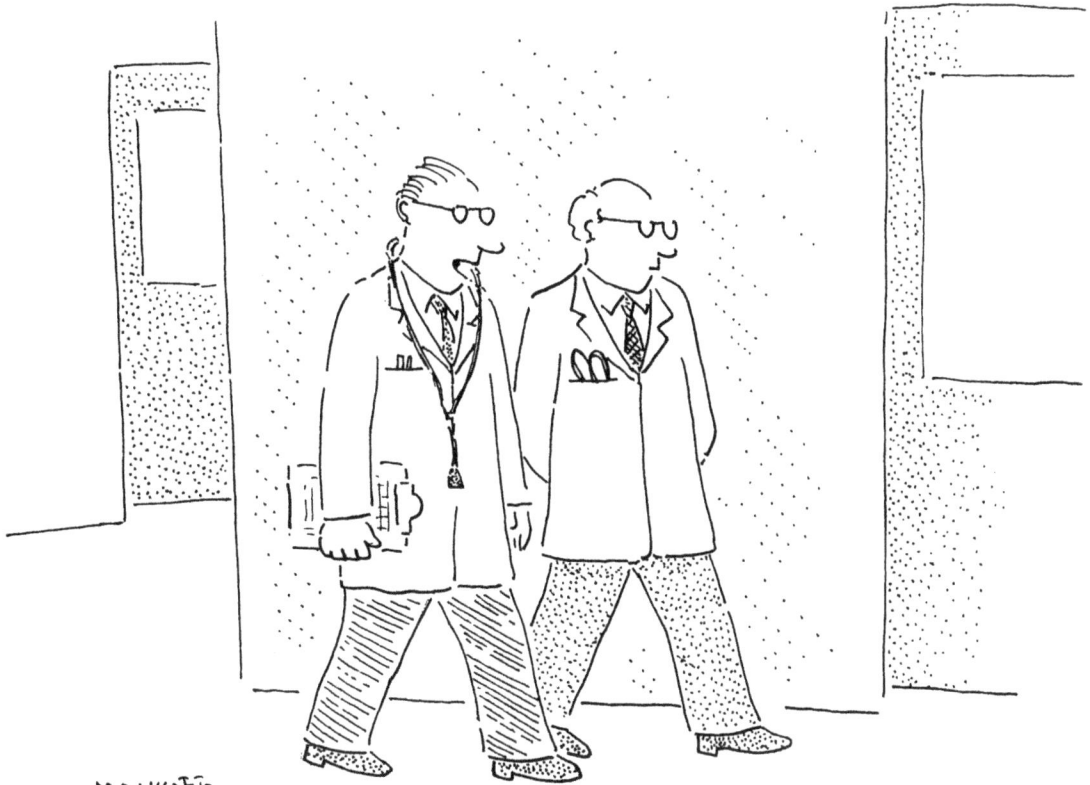

"*I have no objection to alternative medicine so long as traditional medical fees are scrupulously maintained.*"

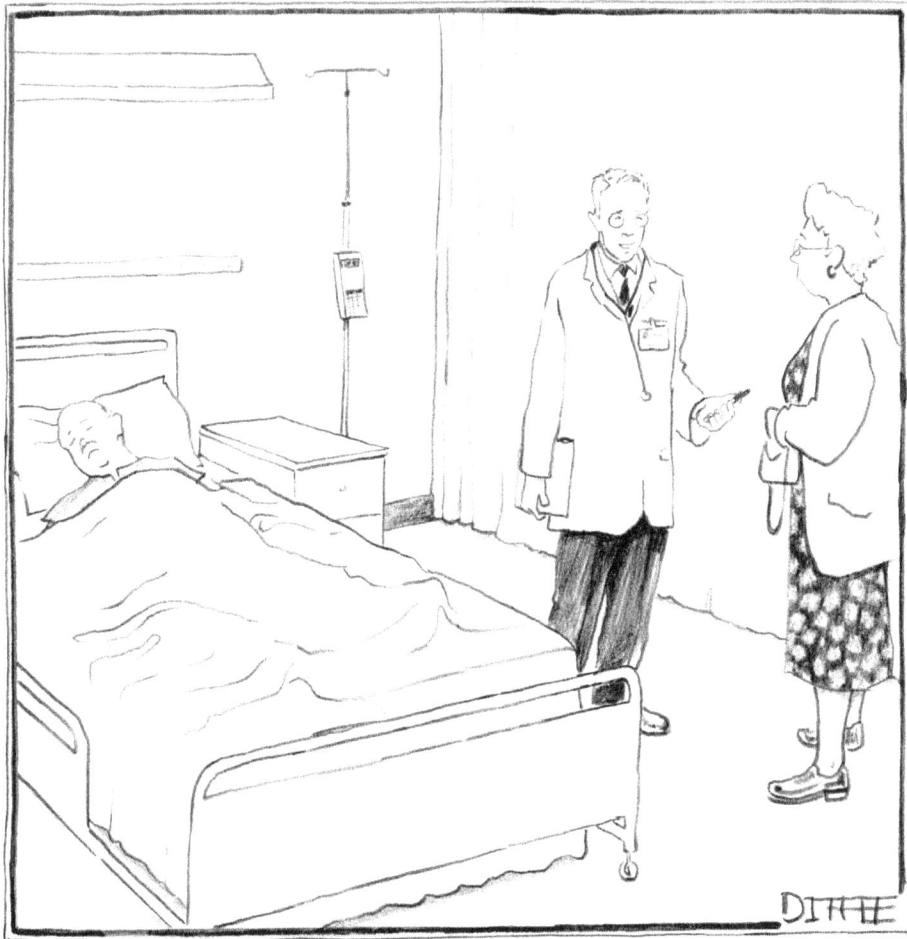

"He's gonna be in and out for a while, so we should
write something funny on his forehead."

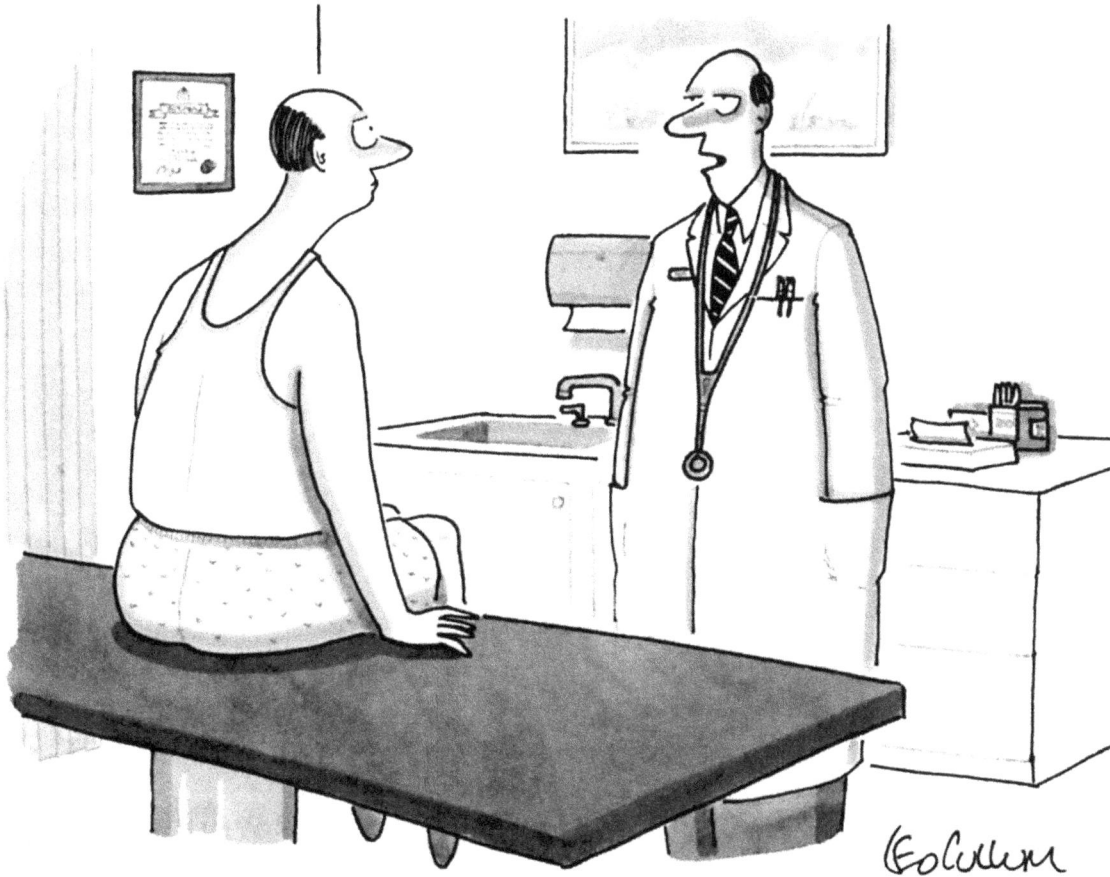

"This is a second opinion. At first, I thought you had something else."

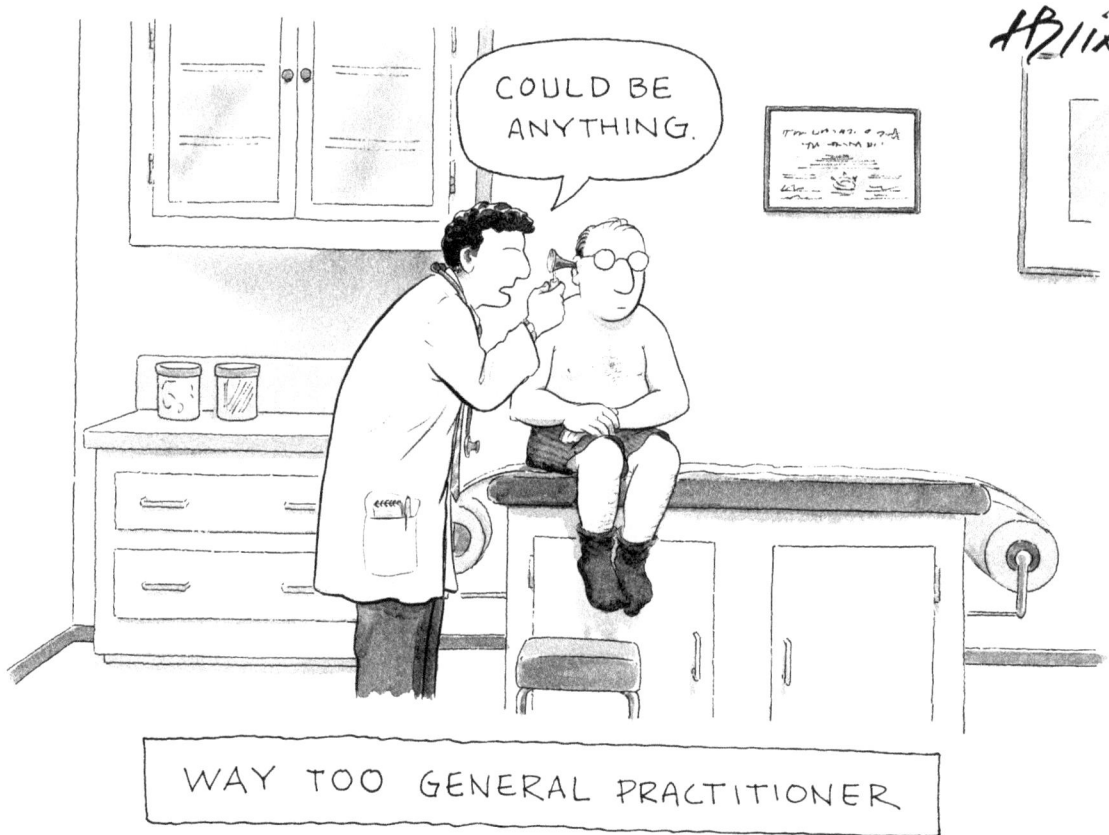

COULD BE ANYTHING.

WAY TOO GENERAL PRACTITIONER

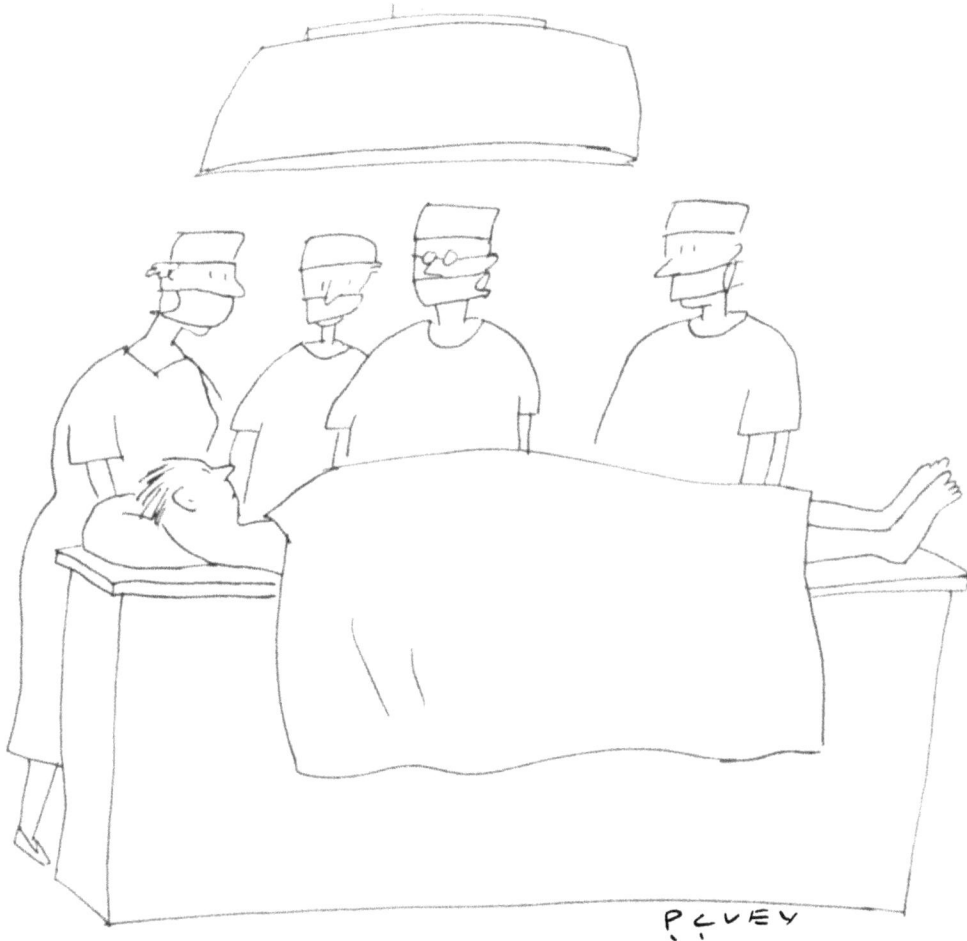

"*Okay - which one of us is talking now?*"

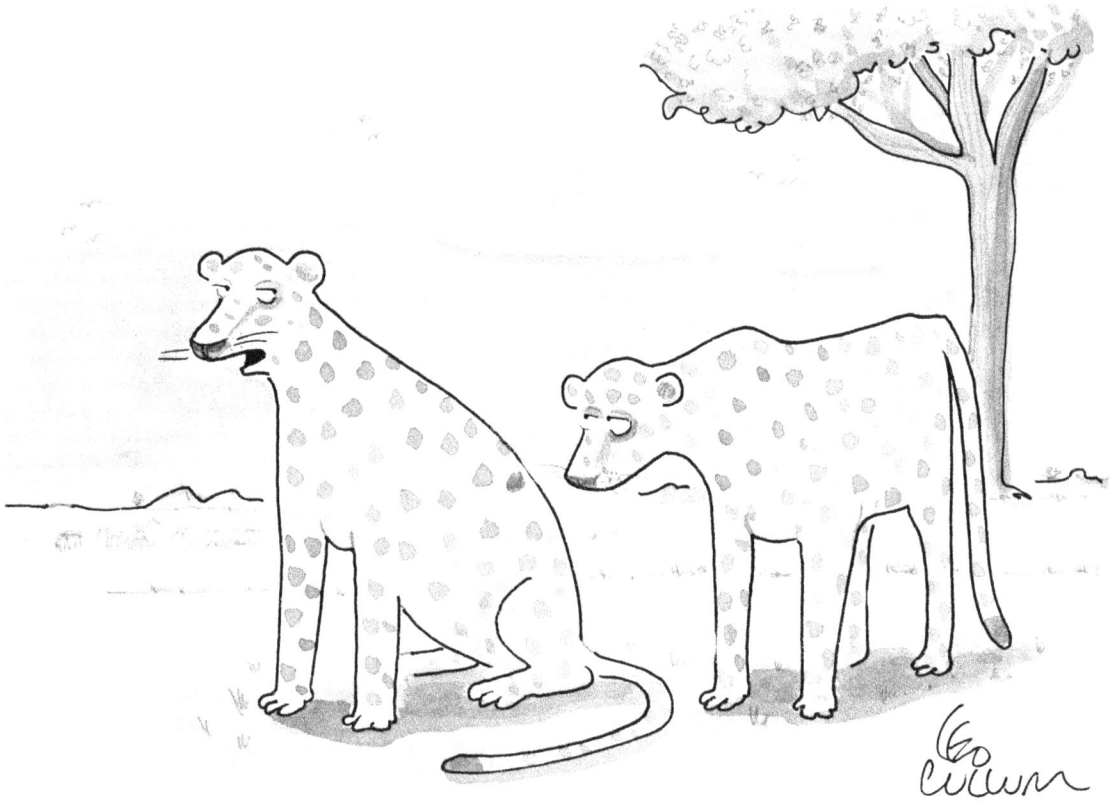

"That one, I think, is a liver spot."

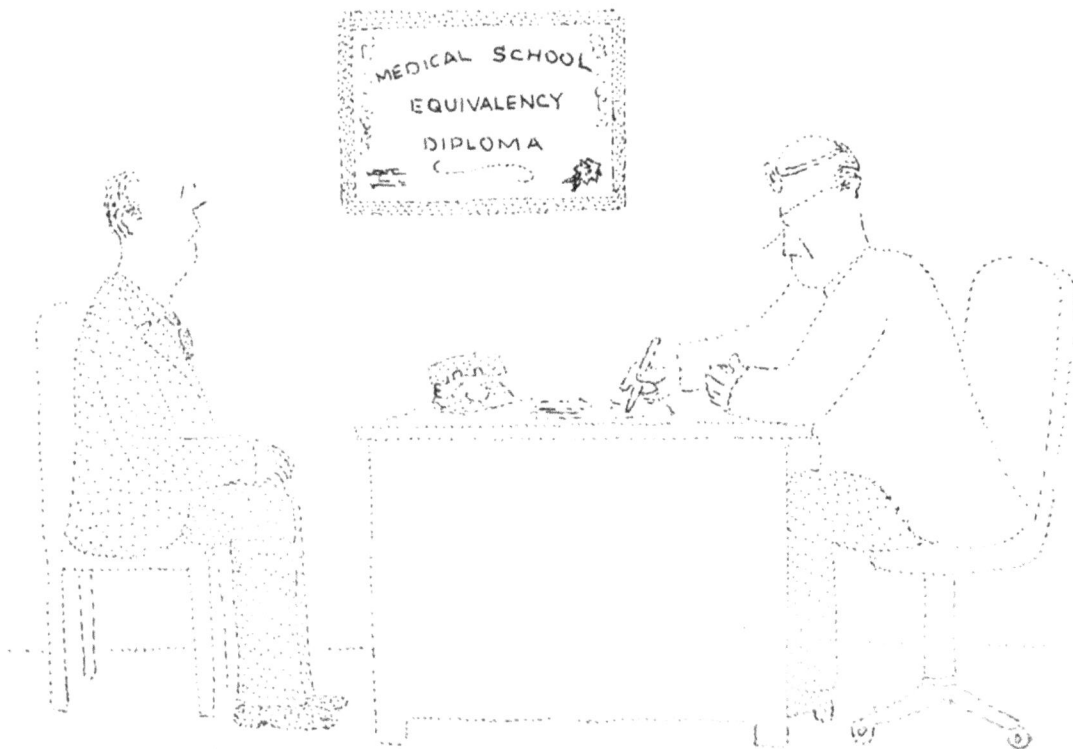

MEDICAL SCHOOL EQUIVALENCY DIPLOMA

MANKOFF

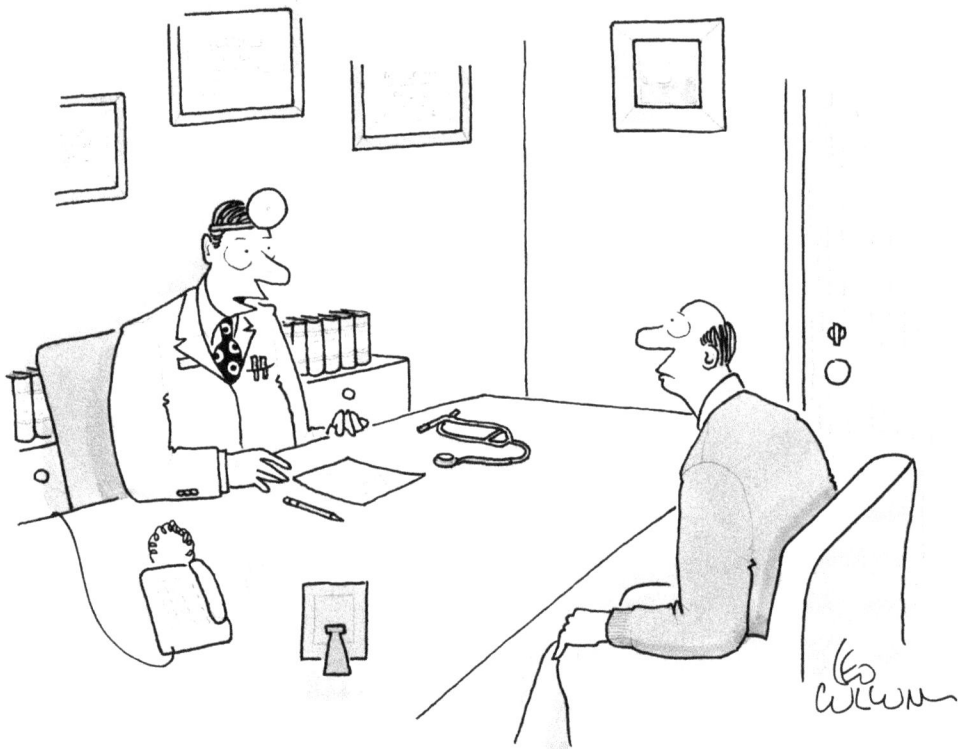

"You have a condition whose name is very hard to remember."

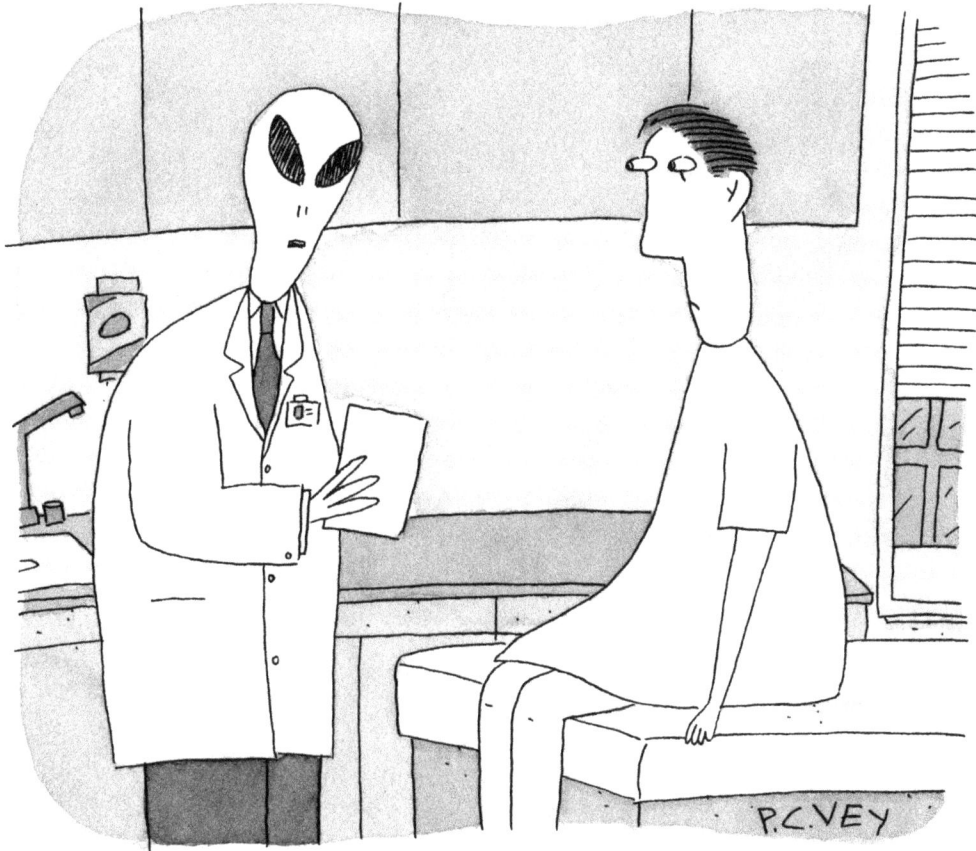

"There's a cure,—but it's light-years away."

Index of Artists

Alex Gregory, 71, 73, 77

Amy Kurzweil, 10, 56

Benjamin Schwartz, 3, 42, 63

Bob Mankoff, 16, 20, 36, 57, 66, 67, 78, 84

Cartoons Hate Her, 25

Charles Barsotti, 26, 50

Charlie Hankin, 13

Chris Wildt, 35

Christopher Weyant, 22, 65

Danny Shanahan, 6, 12, 29, 64, 76

David Sipress, 53

Drew Dernavich, 61

Emily Flake, 75

Frank Cotham, 14

Gahan Wilson, 31

Glen Le Lievre, 68

Harry Bliss, 47, 81

Hilary Campbell, 34

John Grimes, 7

Kaamran Hafeez, 17

Kim Warp, 51

Leo Cullum, 38, 39, 40, 48, 70, 74, 80, 83, 85

Mary Lawton, 43

Matthew Diffee, 79

Mick Stevens, 59

Mike Shapiro, 8

Mike Twohy, 60

P. C. Vey, 18, 21, 37, 52, 69, 82, 86

Pat Byrnes, 11

Paul Noth, 1, 2, 9, 32, 41, 49, 55, 62, 72

Peter Steiner, 4, 28, 44, 46

Rina Piccolo, 54, 58

Robert Leighton, 15, 27, 30

Roz Chast, 5, 19

Sam Gross, 33

Vaughan Tomlinson, 23, 24

Yinfan Huang, 45

www.ingramcontent.com/pod-product-compliance
Lightning Source LLC
Chambersburg PA
CBHW040847100426

42813CB00015B/2736